The
Ultimate HMO
Handbook

The Ultimate HMO Handbook

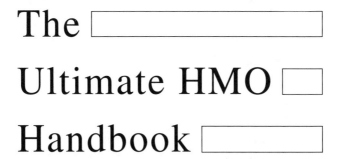

*How to Make the Most from
the Revolution in Managed Care*

Rhys W. Jones, MPH

TTM Health Publishing
Albany, CA

Acknowledgements

The author wishes to give special thanks to the following people for their advice, assistance and suggestions in reviewing *The Ultimate HMO Handbook* during its development:

Robert Barnes	Peggy Grier
Jill Barnes	William Grier
Mara Carli	Jerry Hill
Sara Carnahan	Meredith Jones
Dianne Dobbins	Gerry Jones
Robert Edmondson	Lauren Reffkin

Thanks also to Kathy Billingsley, Zoe Goldman, Caroline Lehman, Ken Stanton, Carol Lee and Chuck Wunderlich

---

The Ultimate HMO Handbook

Copyright © 1994 by TTM Health Publishing

International Standard Book Number: 0-9635819-1-0

Cover art, design and graphics by TTM Health Publishing

Published in the United States of America by TTM Health Publishing, 1070 Neilson Street, Albany, CA 94706. Telephone: (510) 524-4200

Printed in the United States of America.

Table of Contents

Table of Contents

1. Introduction to HMOs

What Are HMOs?

Health maintenance organizations are unique health care organizations that integrate the financing and delivery of health care. Also called *prepaid health plans,* HMOs combine two functions: the same organization provides health coverage to its enrollees or members, and provides them with comprehensive health care services.

There are a number of characteristics that make HMOs unique among health care institutions. An HMO operates in a specific geographic *service area* and is organized around a core group of health care providers called the *provider network.* The HMO provider network is 'built' through contracts with selected physician groups, hospitals and ancillary providers who give the HMO discounts in the anticipation of an increased volume of HMO patients. These selective contracts help HMOs keep prices low while offering care of high quality. HMO enrollees are required to obtain care from these contracting providers, except in cases of emergency (this requirement is sometimes called the *lock-in rule.)*

Unlike traditional insurers, HMOs are actively involved in the care their members receive. They use a variety of managed-care techniques (discussed in Chapter 5) to monitor the quality of care provided, discourage the provision of unnecessary services, and check the credentials of the professionals who provide health services.

As prepaid health plans, HMOs provide health care coverage for a fixed premium paid in advance by the member or employer. From the member's standpoint, there are no financial surprises – all the care the member may need is paid for by the single monthly fee, plus nominal copayments. From the provider's perspective, payments for health services are based on contracted rates that are negotiated in advance.

Traditional health insurance (also known as *indemnity insurance*) pays a certain percentage of the charges billed by the provider, and the patient is responsible for the balance. This method of paying providers is called *fee-for-service*. With fee-for-service, the provider is paid a separate fee for each procedure or service performed.

Unfortunately, paying for health care this way can encourage providers to increase their payments by providing more services of greater complexity. Because HMO care is prepaid and managed, many of the negative financial incentives found in traditional medical care reimbursement are reversed. Prepayment encourages HMOs and their providers to keep enrollees healthy by emphasizing preventive care, health education, and early detection and treatment.

Using a variety of managed-care strategies (see Chapters 2 and 5), HMOs are able to offer health coverage with premiums lower than traditional insurance, while offering enrollees richer benefits and lower out-of-pocket costs. In this way, HMOs make health coverage more affordable and more accessible to employers and their workers. For HMO members, there are other benefits, too. They don't receive bills and aren't required to submit claim forms – under the contractual relationship with the HMO, providers bill the HMO directly.

Who Belongs to HMOs?

Health maintenance organizations are now available in most parts of the United States, with about 540 HMOs operating in 47 states. People enrolled in HMOs are referred to as *members, subscribers* or *enrollees.* In most cases, they join HMOs through an employer's health benefits plan. Others enroll as individuals, converting from group coverage or joining through programs designed to replace Medicare or Medicaid with enhanced benefits.

HMO members come from all sorts of businesses and backgrounds – banking, manufacturing, service industries, school districts, merchant associations, federal, state and municipal governments. These businesses may be of any size, ranging from national employers with thousands of employees to small "mom and pop" businesses. Nearly 20 percent of Americans now receive their care through HMOs, representing a true cross-section of the nation.

HMO Growth Trends

HMOs had approximately 45 million members nationwide at the end of 1993 (see Figure 1 on the next page.) HMO membership has doubled since 1985, and some analysts predict that 25% of all Americans will belong to HMOs by 1996. HMO enrollment varies widely from state to state – in California, over one-third of the population is enrolled in HMOs, while in other states total enrollment may be only a few thousand.

HMOs play a prominent role in a number of national health care reform proposals (see Chapter 10.) Depending on the reform plan implemented, the number of Americans covered by HMOs may increase substantially in the next few years.

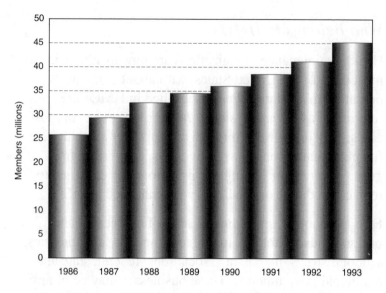

Figure 1. HMO Membership by Year (at year-end)
[Source: GHAA]

HMO Organizational Models

HMOs are organized along several common structures or *models* – staff, group, IPA and network. These models differ primarily in the relationship between the HMO and its physician providers; each model has its own particular set of advantages.

❑ *Staff model* HMOs use physicians who are employed by the HMO itself. Care usually is provided in a clinic facility or medical center owned by the health plan. Staff model HMOs often have lower premiums because they exercise greater control over the provision of health care, thereby minimizing the performance of unnecessary services.

❑ *Group model* plans are formed around a multi-specialty medical group that contracts to provide physician services exclusively to the HMO. Medical group physicians own or are partners of the group, and patients are seen in facilities belonging to either the medical group or the HMO.

❏ *Independent practice association (IPA)* plans are built around a physician association. This is an organization of physicians in private practice who organize for the purpose of contracting with one or more HMOs or insurers. A majority of HMOs are organized along the IPA structure.

In this model, a single contract links the HMO to all of the physicians in the IPA, and HMO enrollees receive care in the IPA physicians' private offices. In practice, as well as in this book, the term *medical group* is often used to refer to any group of physicians organized to contract with managed-care organizations such as HMOs.

❏ *Network model* HMOs contract with a number of IPAs and/or medical groups to form a physician network. This allows an HMO to market its services in a broader geographic area than would be possible with a single physician group.

Another common term, *mixed model HMO,* is used to describe a plan whose provider network consists of a combination of the delivery systems described above, without emphasizing any particular model type. Figure 2 (see next page) shows the relative percentage of HMOs by model type.

Realistically, no single HMO model is right for everybody. Some people like to see their doctor in a traditional medical office, so an IPA-model HMO may be best for them. Others may prefer the convenience of a clinic setting that offers physician services, lab and pharmacy located in a single facility; clinics are more characteristic of group and staff model HMOs. Generally speaking, a network or mixed model offers the widest choice of delivery systems and the broadest geographical coverage.

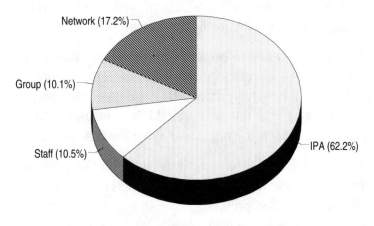

Figure 2. HMOs by Model Type
[Source - GHAA]

Ownership and Control

Like other kinds of health care organizations, HMOs vary widely in *ownership*. Some are owned by publicly-traded, for-profit corporations, while others are operated as charitable or not-for-profit enterprises. Many are single, independent plans operating only in a small geographic area; others are subsidiaries or affiliates of large insurance or managed-care chains with health plans in major cities across the country.

Ownership considerations are of concern to all, but especially to employers who want to make sure that the health plan they choose has good geographic coverage and financial stability. However, enrollees have a vested interest in a plan's *tax status* – not-for-profit vs. for-profit – because tax status may influence an HMO's ability to keep decisions about health care separate from financial considerations.

Government Regulation

HMOs are regulated at the federal level and by state agencies in 47 states. The laws regulating HMOs emphasize access to care, consumer protection and financial stability, and are intended to ensure that plans can deliver on their commitments.

At the federal level, HMOs can voluntarily apply for *federal qualification*. To become federally qualified, the HMO requests a review by a department of the Health Care Financing Administration *(HCFA)*. This federal review evaluates such factors as accessibility of the HMO's provider networks, financial stability, procedures for resolving complaints, management structure, and membership materials. The HMO must also offer a set of mandated benefits (see page 62.)

If the HMO meets these federal requirements, HCFA designates it as *federally qualified*. HMOs seek federal qualification because it is like a government "seal of approval" that makes an HMO more attractive to employers and, therefore, more marketable. In some areas, federal qualification has become less important, but it is still a marketing plus in highly competitive HMO states like California.

At the state level, HMOs must be licensed by an agency such as the Department of Health, Department of Insurance or Department of Corporations. Many state HMO laws are similar to federal qualification regulations and are designed to ensure compliance with minimum standards. Most such laws set minimum requirements for financial viability, compliance with ethical advertising practices, adequacy of administrative resources, accessibility of provider networks, and provision of certain mandated benefits.

State licensure and federal qualification are both given for a specific geographic area called the *service area*. An HMO can market to employer groups and enroll members only within its licensed service area. Service areas are officially designated by county, or by zip code in cases where only a part of a county is served. In contrast, traditional insurers may be licensed to operate in an entire state. Although their employer contracts and benefit plan designs may be regulated, they cannot offer the benefits of contracted provider networks (see Credentialing in Chapter 9.)

Other Forms of Managed Care

Popular as they are, HMOs are not the only forms of managed care available. However, they are the most comprehensive, highly-integrated form of managed-care system, and the most efficient at keeping costs low for members and employers. Other managed-care systems base their provider reimbursements on variations of the fee-for-service method. Therefore, their providers do not share in the financial risks, so they are not as effective at controlling costs as HMOs. Furthermore, these systems place little emphasis on prevention and health maintenance. Other systems include:

❏ *Preferred provider organizations (PPOs)* are arrangements in which an insurer contracts with a group of physicians, hospitals and ancillary providers (the "preferred providers") at discounted rates. PPO coverage provides financial incentives for enrollees to receive services from preferred providers. If services are received from a preferred provider, the PPO covers a greater portion of the cost. If services are received from non-PPO providers, the PPO still covers the services, but at a reduced rate, so the member is required to pay more. Some employers regard

PPOs as a sort of compromise between HMOs and indemnity insurance plans – PPOs provide coverage at some cost savings while allowing the enrollee the option of receiving care from any provider.

From a financial standpoint, the PPO arrangement provides preferred providers with an increased volume of patients in exchange for discounted rates, but the providers have no incentive to control expenses because they have no financial risk. To control utilization, many PPOs include managed-care techniques, such as referral systems, hospital preauthorization and utilization review (see Chapter 5.) However, when used piecemeal, these elements are not as effective as when they are integrated into the comprehensive utilization management programs found in HMOs.

❏ *Managed Indemnity Plans* are traditional insurance plans that have borrowed some of the managed-care techniques used by HMOs (as mentioned above). Provider reimbursement is on a fee-for-service basis, and the insured person is responsible for coinsurance and deductibles (see Chapter 7.) As with PPOs, providers typically have little incentive to control costs. Managed indemnity products are attractive to those who want an unlimited choice of doctors, but such plans are not priced much lower than traditional indemnity plans.

HMO Market Focus

HMOs may differ from each other by the markets on which they focus and in the kinds of people they seek as members. Most plans are *full service HMOs* that offer a comprehensive range of health care services; these HMOs are the focus of this book. Others are called *specialty HMOs,* which offer coverage in a certain health field such as mental health or dental care.

HMOs concentrate foremost on the commercial employer market, providing services to the employees of businesses, unions and governmental bodies. This is by far the largest market with the greatest potential for members and revenue. After becoming established with commercial accounts, many plans expand to offer health coverage to participants in government-financed programs such as Medicare and Medicaid.

In a *Medicare risk HMO* plan, for example, the administration of a member's Medicare coverage and benefits is assumed by the Medicare HMO, with the approval of the member and HCFA. The federal Medicare program pays the HMO a fixed monthly premium to provide all necessary care to the member. This premium is about 5% lower than the average amount Medicare would otherwise spend for care through the fee-for-service system.

The HMO then must provide the member with all of the benefits covered by regular Medicare, and may provide other benefits that Medicare does not cover. In this relationship, there are potential benefits for all concerned – the government program can save money, the enrollee receives coordinated care and enhanced benefits, and the HMO gains membership and revenue. Medicare HMO plans are discussed in detail in Chapter 6.

•

This first chapter has provided a brief overview of HMOs, how they're organized and regulated, their target markets, and how they differ from traditional health insurance plans. With this general background, we will now look at two areas of vital interest to prospective and current HMO members: how HMOs provide medical care, and how members can make the most of being in an HMO.

2. Health Care in HMOs

How Is Care Provided?

When doctor and patient meet in an HMO setting, the care the patient receives is not all that different from care provided through the traditional medical system, except that HMO care is provided through and managed by a formalized structure. HMOs differ most from traditional health insurance in these respects: their direct involvement in patient care, networks of contracted providers and use of managed-care techniques. Also, HMOs emphasize prepayment of care to encourage providers to keep members well and minimize costs when members become sick.

In order to manage care, HMOs distinguish between various kinds of medical care. *Primary care* is the type of routine care needed by most people, and consists of immunizations, check-ups, and the diagnosis, treatment and management of most medical conditions. Primary care is typically obtained from general practitioners, internists, family practice physicians and pediatricians. *Specialty care* is focused care dealing with the diagnosis and treatment of specific, non-routine conditions. This type of care is received from physicians who have received additional training in a particular branch of medicine, such as cardiology or surgery.

Acute care refers to the intensive services provided in inpatient settings, such as hospitals, for serious or complex conditions. *Emergency care* refers to the intensive services given in an emergency room or ambulance which are necessary to stabilize a patient and prevent loss of life or worsening of the patient's condition.

The Role of Physician Organizations

As we mentioned, most HMOs contract with organized groups of physicians to provide professional services to the HMO's members. Physicians form these organizations – known by names such as *independent practice associations (IPAs), group practices,* or *medical groups* – to negotiate and contract with HMOs (especially IPA and network-model plans) and other managed-care organizations. The physician group may also provide its doctors with other advantages, such as volume purchasing arrangements for medical supplies and malpractice insurance. In some cases, a physician group may contract exclusively with one HMO, but many have contracts with several HMOs. In group-model plans, the medical group is often closely allied with the HMO in an exclusive arrangement.

Physician organizations are governed by boards of directors made up of member physicians. An administrative staff oversees day-to-day operations; in the smallest groups, staff may consist of a part-time medical director and a few support personnel, while larger groups may have administrators and dozens of support staff in many departments.

The administrative capabilities of a medical group can vary markedly from group to group. In the smallest groups, the group may rely on an outside source or the HMO itself for claims processing and information system support, while larger groups may have their own claims processing, computer systems and utilization review functions. The strength and sophistication of a medical group are of considerable importance to an HMO in the areas of quality management, effectiveness in controlling costs and the ability of the group's administration to motivate the physicians to work efficiently together as a coordinated network.

Like HMOs, medical groups may subcontract for some health care services, just as HMOs subcontract with them for physician professional services. Almost any service can be subcontracted, such as laboratory, anesthesia services, utilization review, mental health or physical therapy. Subcontractors may be individual providers or other organized provider groups, but the important distinction is that they are not a part of the medical group and are not directly under the medical group's control. Fortunately, however, these administrative arrangements are transparent to most members. The individual member receives care from individual physicians and providers, relatively unaware of the contractual structure through which they may be organized.

The Primary Care Physician

With traditional insurance coverage, people are not restricted from receiving their routine medical care from specialist physicians. However, this situation encourages a patchwork approach to medical care which is quite expensive; care from multiple physicians frequently results in the duplication of services and the provision of services that are inappropriate. Furthermore, there is seldom any coordination of the treatments received from different physicians, and the treatments can interfere with each other and may even be dangerous to the patient.

Most HMOs resolve this problem by requiring that each enrollee select a *primary care physician (PCP)* to serve as his or her personal doctor. Using PCPs provides several important benefits. The patient is encouraged to establish a relationship with the primary physician; this allows the physician to get to know the patient and the patient's medical history. The physician is then in a position to coordinate the patient's care more effectively.

The PCP also serves as a *gatekeeper* who provides the member with day-to-day routine care, and allows the patient access to more expensive specialty care only when necessary. Of course, this keeps costs lower, but consider also that medical procedures are among those things in life where *more* does not necessarily mean *better.* The gatekeeper approach has the added benefit of minimizing the provision of unnecessary or duplicated services, either of which increase the patient's chances of complications.

Is Choice Really An Issue?

Critics of HMOs often charge that the choice of physicians in HMOs is too restricted, and imply that only the traditional health care system offers the individual a real choice without limitations. But does traditional fee-for-service medical care really offer unlimited choice?

As health care consumers, choosing a family doctor is the single most important health care decision that most of us will ever make. While the choice may be based on a number of factors, people don't always appreciate that the choice has far-reaching effects. The choice of physician may be based largely on immediate concerns, such as training, office location, bedside manner or reputation, but the decision also determines the hospitals to which one may be admitted, and the specialists and other providers from whom one will receive other kinds of care.

Physicians develop a *pattern of practice* – an informal network of specialists to whom they make referrals and two or three hospitals where they admit their patients. They routinely refer patients to specific laboratories, pharmacies and ancillary providers, and build relationships with the physicians in their after-hours on-call groups.

It is clear that in choosing a family doctor and becoming subject to his or her pattern of practice, the individual must then accept that the doctor effectively limits the patient's choice of other possible providers. These limitations affect people regardless of whether their care is paid for through an HMO or by traditional insurance. Therefore, the assertion that HMOs limit their members' choice of providers must be viewed in this context.

While HMO enrollees must choose from among an HMO's participating providers, many HMOs – especially IPA and network plans – have provider networks that offer members a choice from among hundreds of PCPs. HMO members make an additional choice when they choose a primary care physician who is part of a medical group or IPA. In such cases, the choice of specialists to whom the PCP can routinely refer patients may be limited to those who are members of the same medical group as the PCP.

Tips on Choosing a Primary Care Physician

While choosing a PCP might seem to be easy, making a good choice takes some work, and you'll find that doing a little research will pay off. Start by asking the HMO for a copy of its physician directory. In network and IPA-model HMOs, provider directories often are designed to make it easy to find physicians by location, and many have special sections of physicians with second language capabilities. Ask the HMO's Member Services department to give you the names of several PCPs in your area. Group and staff-model HMOs may have special physician directories for each facility. One of your best bets is word of mouth – ask any friends or colleagues who are covered by the HMO for their PCP recommendations.

Consider the doctor relationship that is most important to you. Do you want one doctor to care for your whole family? If so, try a family practice physician. Family practitioners undergo a three-year residency in which they receive specialized training in general and internal medicine, pediatrics, and obstetrics and gynecology. Upon completion of the residency, they are eligible to take a certification examination of the American Board of Family Practice. Family practice physicians are well qualified to provide comprehensive, routine care for the entire family.

Some people may want a physician in a more traditional specialty. Will the HMO allow you to choose a pediatrician for your children and an internist for yourself? Is bedside manner more important, or familiarity with the latest medical advances? Ideally, you'll want a balance between the two. A doctor who has recently completed a residency and board certification will score high on technical knowledge, but an older physician will have more experience and perspective. Consider other characteristics that may be important to you. Do you prefer a male or a female physician? Do you have any special language needs? Would you prefer a physician located near home or close to work?

Prepare a list of several suitable candidates – some doctors are so popular that they may not be accepting new patients. If you're in a network or IPA HMO, contact each physician's office and explain that you're looking for a family doctor and would like some information. Find out the names of the hospitals where the doctor admits patients. Which other physicians share in the doctor's on-call group? In how many other HMOs does the physician participate? How long has he or she been in practice?

Stop by the office – note the office hours, the mood of the office staff and mood of the patients in the waiting room. Does the staff seem courteous and well organized? Are the patients unhappy because they've been waiting too long? If you're just getting into an HMO but already have a family doctor, ask your doctor if he or she is part of the HMO provider network or has any plans to join. If not, ask if he or she can recommend any of the physicians in the HMO's physician network.

Most importantly, you should be comfortable with the PCP relationship. A good primary care physician should be responsive to your questions, respectful of your wishes and sensitive to your feelings. Your primary care physician is someone you are going to have to trust and work with to maintain your health. Most HMOs will allow you to change PCPs several times until you find one you're satisfied with. When you make a selection, try the new doctor out for a while. It may take a few tries to find a PCP you're happy with, but it's worth it in the long run.

Changing PCPs

In many HMOs, changing your primary care physician can be done by simply notifying the HMO that you wish to change. Each HMO has its own particular policy regarding PCP changes – some allow changes by telephone, but many require advance written notification. Some plans will allow you to change as often as you wish, while others limit the number of changes to once or twice per year (this may be negotiable for good cause.) When you change, be ready to inform the HMO of your new PCP choice. If you have trouble choosing, contact the HMO's Member Service department for help. In most plans, PCP changes become effective the first of the month following the request.

Making Appointments

After joining an HMO, the process of obtaining routine primary care changes very little, except for the fact that care must be obtained through the PCP. In IPA and network model plans, the member simply calls the primary care physician's office to schedule an appointment. In staff and group models, the member's call may be taken by a central appointment line which makes appointments for all physicians in the facility. The appointment is normally made with the member's PCP, but the patient may be seen by any available physician for urgent care or in HMOs where PCPs are not assigned. A copayment is often charged for the visit, and is paid when checking in with the receptionist.

Receiving care from specialists is quite different in HMOs. As noted previously, members usually cannot self-refer for specialty care. Instead, the member must first call or visit his or her PCP for an initial evaluation. If the PCP feels that specialty care is required, the PCP will give the patient a formal referral to a specialist (for more on Referrals, see Chapter 5.) The specialist chosen by the PCP may work for the HMO exclusively or have a private practice in the community. In any event, he or she has a contract with the HMO or physician group to provide services to HMO patients.

Once the referral is made, the patient contacts the specialist's office to make an appointment. The specialist sees the patient, evaluates the patient's condition, and then reports findings and recommended treatments to the PCP for follow-up. While the patient may pay a small copayment, the bill for the specialist's consultation is paid by either the HMO or the medical group (see Chapter 8.)

Telephone Advice Lines

Some larger HMOs offer telephone-based *advice lines* to help members decide whether their symptoms require medical attention. Advice lines are most common in staff and group-model HMOs, and are usually operated by registered nurses working under the supervision of staff physicians.

The main job of the advice nurse is to help the patient separate urgent or routine problems from emergencies. After talking with the patient and reviewing the patient's symptoms, the nurse can usually recommend the appropriate course of action. The patient may be advised to wait and see if his or her symptoms continue, be given an urgent-care appointment for later on the same day, or be directed to an emergency room for immediate treatment of serious conditions.

Of course, advice lines are used by HMOs to control and decrease the demand for access to same-day appointments and urgent care services. However, advice lines also perform a valuable service for members. Advice nurses provide the personalized attention, information and reassurance that many people need, whether to new parents who are unsure about a symptom their baby may be having or to an elderly member concerned about a new medication.

Emergency Services

Emergency care is the one circumstance in which HMO members may receive care from a non-plan provider without prior authorization. Most HMOs establish policies that distinguish between emergency treatment within the plan's service area and treatment received outside the service area *(out-of-area care)*. The member or provider must notify the HMO as soon as possible after treatment has been given. This allows the HMO to involve its providers in the clinical management of the case or arrange for transfer to a participating facility.

Within the service area, the HMO encourages enrollees to contact their PCP when urgent medical attention is needed. This permits the PCP to assess the patient's condition, determine whether the patient should be seen in the office or the emergency room, and direct the member to a contracting facility if needed. If the patient's condition prevents him or her from contacting the PCP prior to treatment, the member or treating hospital is requested to contact the HMO as soon as possible after care is given. Of course, in a *bona fide* emergency, treatment is covered even if it is not provided by a contracting facility.

Outside of the HMO's service area, emergency services from any provider are covered, provided that an emergency existed. Some plans may not cover out-of-area emergency treatment for conditions that could have been reasonably foreseen by the enrollee, but this is not the rule.

Emergency claims may be subject to review by the HMO prior to payment. The purpose of these reviews is to confirm that the patient's condition required emergency treatment, and that the enrollee was not seen for some minor or chronic complaint, such as a cold. If the HMO finds that the patient's condition clearly didn't require emergency treatment, the HMO may deny the claim and the patient will be financially responsible for the services.

In the emergency room, an HMO enrollee is treated the same as any other patient. ER staff will record basic patient information and a brief description of the patient's problem. They will also request insurance information, any applicable copayment, and a copy of the enrollee's HMO membership card. With this information in hand, the emergency staff will contact the HMO to verify eligibility and obtain coverage information. In life-threatening emergencies where the HMO enrollee cannot provide information, hospitals in most states are required to treat and stabilize the patient and ask questions later. The hospital can contact the HMO afterwards to resolve any eligibility or administrative issues.

Hospital Care

The use of hospital services is the aspect of medical care most tightly controlled by HMOs. As hospital care is the most expensive form of treatment for many illnesses, HMOs require that all hospital services proposed for an enrollee be reviewed in advance and authorized by the HMO and the PCP's medical group if applicable (see Chapter 5.)

Although group and staff HMOs often operate their own hospitals, they frequently contract with medical centers and teaching hospitals to provide certain specialized procedures, such as heart surgery and transplants. IPA and network HMOs provide hospital care by contracting with several key hospitals in a given geographic area for acute hospital services. In such contractual relationships, the hospital gives the HMO discounted rates in exchange for an increased volume of patients and prompt payment of bills. HMOs negotiate contracts with the most popular and established hospitals in a community because having these hospitals in the network makes the HMO more attractive to enrollees and more marketable to employers.

For the average HMO member, a hospital admission is no different than for a person covered by traditional indemnity insurance. After the HMO authorizes the admission, the admitting physician contacts the hospital to reserve a room and schedule needed procedures. On arrival, the patient is interviewed by a representative of the hospital's Admitting department to obtain personal and financial information.

Once admitted, the patient receives the same care as any other patient, but with a few differences. Behind the scenes, the patient's care is reviewed regularly by the HMO to confirm the ongoing need for hospitalization (see Utilization Review in Chapter 5.) In IPA and network plans, HMO staff may confer regularly with the attending physician concerning the patient's status and the plans for follow-up care when the patient goes home. After discharge, the hospital bill is sent to the HMO for processing and payment. The member's financial responsibility is limited to any applicable copayments and charges for non-covered hospital services, such as television and guest meals. In staff and group-model HMOs where the HMO operates the hospital facility, utilization review takes place as an in-house function, and the billing function is concerned with accounting for expenses instead of billing the patient's insurance.

Home Care

HMOs provide a variety of medical services in the home, in situations where home care offers a viable alternative to hospital admission. This approach is especially beneficial to the patient because he or she can recuperate at home in familiar surroundings without the hazards and indignities of institutional care. Services commonly provided in the home setting include home nursing care, physical and speech therapy, and even intravenous drug therapy. In most plans, case managers from the HMO monitor the patient's progress and assist the primary care physician in coordinating treatments and services whenever several home care providers are involved (see page 56.) Larger staff and group-model HMOs may operate their own home care departments; most network and IPA plans contract for services from community-based agencies or visiting nurse associations.

Health Promotion

HMOs offer health promotion and education programs to their members. While programs are required by many states, most HMOs actively support them because they encourage members to adopt healthier lifestyles and to take an active role in prevention.

Programs vary widely in scope and complexity, depending on a plan's size and resources. Many programs provide health education classes, materials on how to reduce risk factors (for example, how to lower cholesterol or quit smoking); and programs on infant care and child safety. Some plans arrange discounted memberships for their enrollees at health clubs and fitness centers. Health promotion is another way that HMOs keep their commitment to maintaining the health of their members.

Other Services

HMOs provide comprehensive health services to their members through HMO facilities or through contracts with providers in the community. Prescription drugs may be furnished through in-house pharmacies (staff and group model HMOs) or through a combination of chain and independent drug stores (IPA and network models).

HMOs contract with private ambulance services or hospitals for emergency transportation. Services from physical, speech and other rehabilitation therapists may be provided by HMO staff, or through medical group providers and therapists in private practice. Opticians and optometrists are often found in-house in staff and group model plans, while most IPA and network plans use the services of community-based optical providers.

•

An HMO actively seeks the participation of selected providers in its networks so that it can offer the full range of medical and health care services through contracted relationships. This increases the HMO's marketability, and its influence on the quality and cost of care provided to its members.

3. Getting The Most From Your HMO

Having read this much of *The Ultimate HMO Handbook,* you now have some understanding of how HMOs are organized and how they provide health care. But what does it really mean to be an HMO member? What advantages do HMOs offer to their members? What are the drawbacks?

If you are considering joining an HMO, you already have some of the theoretical background you need in order to make that choice. But this chapter takes you in a different direction – we'll try to balance some of the theory with some practical guidelines that can help you make the most of your experience. Here, you'll learn how to use the HMO to your best advantage.

HMOs are successful because HMO members have lower out-of-pocket costs, lower premiums and less financial risk compared to traditional insurance (see Chapter 7.) HMOs offer their members richer benefits, especially in the area of preventive services (see Benefits in Chapter 6), and comprehensive care enhanced by quality management and provider credentialing programs (discussed in Chapter 9.)

However, HMO members take greater responsibility for their own care. They give up the unrestricted choice of the fee-for-service system, and the freedom to be frivolous and inefficient in obtaining health care. There are more policies and rules to follow and understand. Treatment decisions are no longer made solely by the patient's physician, but may be made with the participation of the patient, the medical group and the HMO.

Frankly, HMOs work by placing an additional layer of bureaucracy onto the medical care delivery system. As with any bureaucracy, this means that the HMO member must sometimes be more assertive and act as his or her own advocate. HMOs are systems, and people are happiest with their HMOs when they *learn how to work the system.*

What kinds of people should join an HMO? Those who are willing to learn to use an HMO's system. People who want first-rate medical care but don't want to spend a lot of money, especially those with large families. People who want to be more involved in their own health care.

What kind of person *shouldn't* join an HMO? A person with a strong, established relationship with a particular physician, if the physician does not participate in an HMO. Someone who feels that he or she can't adapt to a system with more structure. A person who simply is not comfortable with the idea of managed care. Increasingly, though, people find that HMOs offer state-of-the-art medical care with a combination of low price and high quality.

Ten Key Criteria For Choosing an HMO

When it comes time to choose an HMO, one can think of many factors to consider. Of course, the relative importance of each factor will vary with the individual but, in any event, a good decision requires good information. Good information and careful consideration of your needs are the two necessary elements of a good choice.

Much of the information you'll want from an HMO can be obtained by calling its Member Services department. But what questions should you ask? The following are ten essential criteria to consider in choosing an HMO. While no single HMO will be optimal in every respect, these criteria form a basis for comparing different plans and helping you decide what's important for you. The ten key criteria are:

1. Provider Network and Service Area. For IPA and network model plans, examine a copy of the HMO's provider directory. Does the plan offer a strong provider network in your community? Does it provide you with a good selection of physicians? Are the principal hospitals in your community included in the network? For staff and group model HMOs, how conveniently located is the site where you will receive your routine care? Where would you be seen for emergency or urgent care, if needed? Are laboratory, x-ray and pharmacy facilities located on the premises or do you have to go somewhere else?

Regardless of model type, consider two other service area factors: If you have a child away at school, does the HMO's service area extend to where he or she lives? Also, if you live in one area and work in another, does the HMO permit you to receive routine care in either location?

2. Consumer Rankings. Look for surveys that compare the plan you're considering with other HMOs operating in the same geographic area. Such surveys are often conducted annually by local consumer groups or business publications. Ask the HMO for a copy of its latest member satisfaction survey results. Has the plan produced an "HMO report card" evaluating its performance?

3. Word of Mouth. Talking with someone who has experience with the HMO can provide you with valuable insight. Ask around – how do people feel about the HMO? Ask anyone you know who is a plan member. Ask physicians with whom you may be acquainted what they think of the HMO or what they hear from their colleagues.

4. Plan Size. The number of members that belong to an HMO is an indicator of the HMO's relative financial strength and its ability to remain viable in a competitive market. Try to find out whether membership results from sales growth or from an acquisition (e.g., a merger). A plan that grows through sales based on the service it provides may well be better organized and, therefore, a better choice than a plan that reaches a similar size through acquisitions.

5. Choice of PCPs. Will the HMO allow you to choose a different PCP for each family member, or does it require that all family members receive care from the same physician? Can family members each choose a PCP from a different medical group? Decide what's important for you, then keep it in mind as you compare HMOs.

6. Costs and Benefits. Copayments are the major out-of-pocket expense for most HMO members. Review a Summary Plan Description for the type of coverage you would have. Are the copayments reasonable for the services you would use most often? Keep in mind that fixed copayments are more advantageous than coinsurance based on a percentage of charges (see Chapter 7.) Also, if you have to pay a portion of the premium, remember to add in your contribution amount for each plan. Try to determine which HMO will provide the best care for the least cost.

7. Company Characteristics. Find out about the company that owns the HMO. Is it a managed-care company or does it run the HMO as a sideline? How long has it been in business? How much experience does it have with HMOs? How is its recent financial performance? Is it a for-profit or non-profit corporation? For-profit plans may be more restrictive in interpreting benefits and coverage issues because they may be more concerned with profitability and maintaining value for their stockholders.

8. Quality of Care. What percentage of the plan's participating physicians are board-eligible or board-certified? Does the HMO verify the credentials of its physicians, hospitals and other providers? Does the plan use the National Practitioner Data Bank to check on disciplinary and legal actions involving its physicians? For bonus points: has the HMO been accredited by the National Commission on Quality Assurance? (see Accreditation in Chapter 9.)

9. Disenrollment Rates and Reasons. Try asking the HMO's Membership Services representative for information on disenrollment rates of people who voluntarily quit the plan, and the reasons most often given for disenrollment. While many plans don't make this information public, it's worth a try because disenrollment data can tell you a lot about a plan. A low rate of disenrollment indicates that members are satisfied with the service provided. Reasons such as "moved out of town", "got married" and "changed jobs" do not indicate a service problem. On the other hand, watch for reasons such as "not enough doctors", "the plan doesn't pay my bills on time" and "I can't get an appointment" – responses like these may be signs of trouble.

10. Commitment to Customer Service. In the course of researching the HMO, what impressions have you developed? Have staff been courteous and responsive to your requests for information? How does the plan handle phone calls – is it easy to navigate through the phone system to talk with a real person? When you talked with the Membership Services department, did they seem knowledgeable and well-organized? If you have ongoing or special medical needs, does the HMO have any special programs from which you could benefit?

Working The System

This section presents some tips on how to get the most from your HMO. First, and most important, become familiar with your HMO's basic rules and procedures. They are explained in a booklet – the *Summary Plan Description,* as we'll call it in this book (other names include *Coverage Certificate* and *Evidence of Coverage).* Your HMO will give you one when you first enroll. Be sure to review all of your enrollment materials and discuss them with your spouse so you both understand how they apply to your family's situation. For most people, after this important step, being an HMO member simply becomes a matter of going to the doctor and obtaining care when needed.

Planning Your Care

Once you join an HMO and select a PCP, don't stop there – lay out a personal health care network before you need it. Use the HMO provider directory to map out the health resources you're most likely to use, considering your health needs and those of your family.

Determine the locations of the most convenient participating hospital, emergency facility, clinical laboratory and pharmacy. If you have a chronic condition that requires occasional care from a specialist, try to locate several candidates nearby who belong to your PCP's physician group. With this information, you're prepared to state your preferences when your PCP refers you for specialty care.

Consider making a health care journal for yourself. This is a small notebook that you use to record the details of your encounters with the medical system. It's an excellent method for keeping your medical history. Use it to record visit dates, the doctor's name, symptoms, treatments and questions. It may seem a bit compulsive, but it can provide you with valuable information and better understanding of your health. It's also a good place to carry your HMO membership card and copayment receipts.

After joining an HMO and deciding on a primary care physician, begin to establish the relationship. It's important to get to know your PCP so that you're not a total stranger the first time you really need care. Many new HMO members begin their relationship by seeing their new physician for a history and physical exam. This approach gives your new doctor baseline information on your health status, and begins to build the relationship between the two of you.

When You Need Care

• If you have immunization books or height/weight books for your children, bring them along every time your children see the doctor.

• Before your doctor appointment, write down any questions you would like answered so you don't forget them during your consultation.

• Some kinds of appointments, especially routine physicals and gynecologic exams, take more of the doctor's time and require longer booking lead times (scheduling in advance). Keep in mind that you may need to schedule such appointments one to two months ahead.

• If you contact your HMO or PCP after hours or on weekends, you'll probably get the doctor's answering service. Sometimes they need to verify your HMO eligibility, so have your HMO member ID number ready. Also, try to avoid calling late at night – you'll get better service when people are awake.

• Try to schedule appointments for early in the day or right after lunch. The doctor is more likely to be on schedule and you shouldn't have to wait as long because of emergencies and urgent patients. Also, Fridays and Mondays are busy days, with people preparing for or recovering from the weekend. Try to avoid these days and schedule your appointment on a Tuesday, Wednesday or Thursday.

• If you belong to an HMO that has an advice or urgent care line, call the line before making an urgent care appointment. You may save yourself an unnecessary trip.

• Double-check with your physician and/or office staff to ensure that any necessary referrals or authorizations have been obtained prior to obtaining secondary care.

Avoiding Administrative Headaches

• Know and follow your HMO's referral and authorization procedures.

• Carry your HMO identification card with you at all times. Having the card with you when you need it can avoid all sorts of administrative hassles later on.

• Your HMO plan's benefits and rules are explained in the Summary Plan Description. Be a smart consumer – this is your rule book, so study it and get to know your benefits and your HMO's administrative procedures.

• Ask about your HMO's copayment policy. Most HMOs have a policy that you pay only one copayment per office visit, even if you receive several services. Also, ask about office visit copayments for non-physician services, such as follow-up blood pressure checks by a nurse.

• Always get a receipt when you pay a copayment. Save your receipts for one year, just in case.

- If you have a benefit plan with high copayments, especially for hospital admissions, find out about your plan's annual out-of-pocket maximum and keep track of your copayments (see Chapter 6.)

- If you make any payments directly to the HMO, such as premiums for an individual plan, always pay by check or money order and get a receipt. Indicate on the check the months for which you are paying.

- If you change PCPs or medical groups, change your address, or add or drop a dependent from coverage, always notify the HMO in writing and keep a copy. This way, you have a record of what you told your HMO, and can provide the HMO with a duplicate if they lose the original. You don't need to resort to certified mail, but note on your copy the date you mail the notification to your HMO.

- Many HMOs use so-called "automated attendant" computer systems to answer telephone calls. These systems can make call handling more efficient by routing calls to an available staff person. However, this is not always the case – some systems are poorly designed or implemented. If you have repeated problems with long waits on the telephone, by all means COMPLAIN. And remember – most systems allow you the option of avoiding the automated system and having your call handled by a human receptionist.

Solving Problems and Resolving Disputes

Most people don't want to think about the possibility of having problems with their health coverage. And in truth, most HMO members don't have problems with their HMOs. However, should a problem arise, you're in a better position to reach a satisfactory resolution if you understand the procedures your plan uses to resolve problems.

HMOs are complex organizations, and their very complexity can be a source of problems for members, providers and HMOs themselves. This section presents some strategies for presenting your case and resolving problems to your satisfaction.

Seven Rules for Effective Complaints

1. Know The Rules of the Game. Read your Summary Plan Description to refamiliarize yourself with the HMO policies relevant to your situation.

2. Summarize the Situation. Prepare a one paragraph summary, describing in simple terms the problem you are having and how you believe the problem should be resolved. Use the summary when you call the HMO or write a letter.

3. Document Events. Prepare a brief chronology of events pertaining to the problem. This will help you organize your story and can be a useful reference when you contact or write the HMO.

4. Communicate Effectively. Be calm and clear in presenting your problem to the HMO. Your goal is to make them understand and persuade them to correct the problem to your satisfaction. Use relevant portions of the plan summary and your chronology to make your case.

5. Document Contacts. Contact your HMO's Member Services department, using your summary to describe the problem. Keep a record of the date and time of your conversation, and the name and phone number of the person with whom you have contact.

6. Insist on Specifics. When a resolution is promised, ask the Member Services representative for details. If an explanation is not clear, ask for clarification until it makes sense. Ask by what date the problem will be resolved, and whom you should contact for any remaining problems. An acknowledgement of your complaint should come within 15 days, although final resolution may take longer.

7. Use the System. Be persistent and use the grievance and appeals processes (see page 107.) In many HMOs, these processes include binding arbitration as the last step. In most disputes, assistance from an attorney is not necessary, but you may wish to contact one if other attempts at resolution have failed.

Other Problem Solving Strategies

Always let the HMO know if you experience billing or service problems with a provider or medical group. The HMO provider specialists are best equipped to deal with these issues, and you may be doing yourself and others a favor by bringing it to their attention.

When trying to resolve a problem or accomplish some administrative goal, remember that, like any other complex organization, HMOs are bureaucratic. Be assertive without being pushy – your task is to make the HMO representative understand the nature of your problem. Stay focused on the problem – you'll be more persuasive and effective if you keep descriptions brief and to the point.

If you write a complaint letter to your HMO, remember that you are trying to persuade someone to accept your point of view. Read your Summary Plan Description so that you are familiar with the rules and policies applicable to your complaint. Structure the tone of your letter so that you appear to be serious, determined and knowledgeable. Above all, you don't want to appear to be a "crackpot";

most of the time, sending copies of your letter to the President or the Governor is not going to help your case, nor is it usually necessary. However, a letter to the president of the HMO can be quite effective.

Make the HMO's grievance process your main resource. This avoids the unnecessary expense and delay that may result if you complain through a lawyer or regulatory agency, and ensures that your grievance is heard by the appropriate management of the HMO. You can always use lawyers and regulatory agencies if the grievance system proves to be unsatisfactory.

Even though you may have established some helpful contacts in various HMO departments, it's best to route any problems through the Member Services department. Member Services staff are trained to serve as advocates for plan members and have tracking systems to monitor the status of complaints and grievances.

In many HMOs, a letter is sufficient to initiate a formal grievance proceeding. However, some HMOs require that members complete a special grievance form to file a formal complaint. Make sure you understand the plan's rules for filing formal complaints.

If you feel you're getting the runaround when trying to resolve a problem, let your employer know. Quite often, if the employer contacts the HMO group service representative, the service representative can accomplish a resolution. After all, the HMO wants to keep its employer groups satisfied so they will continue to renew their plan coverage each year.

If you get into a serious dispute with your HMO and feel that, despite your efforts, the HMO is not being responsive, find out who the regulators are and give them a call.

At the state level, this may be the Department of Insurance, Health, Corporations or Consumer Affairs. For members of Medicare HMOs, there are specific grievance and appeal procedures which apply (see page 109.) Regional offices of the Health Care Financing Administration (HCFA) can provide you with further information and assistance.

•

One final note on resolving problems. Even though the HMO may have caused a problem, treat the HMO staff politely and cordially. Remember that the HMO representative on the other end of the phone probably does want to help. The person you're talking with probably didn't create your problem. He or she has feelings, too, and people are more responsive to a courteous manner. By encouraging cooperation, you stand a better chance of successfully reaching your objective.

4. Becoming an HMO Member

This chapter examines some of the "behind the scenes" activities involved in enrolling people as HMO members – how HMO coverage is presented and sold to the employer, how eligibility policies are administered, and how members are enrolled and begin to receive care.

Selling the Product and the Plan

Let's first examine some of the factors involved in marketing and selling HMO coverage. When an employer shops for health coverage, he or she looks for several things: good benefits, a wide choice of providers, a service area that meets the needs of employees, and responsive service – all at a reasonable price. For its part, the HMO is interested in enrolling groups that have average levels of medical utilization and will yield a reasonable profit.

The sales process begins when the employer calls the HMO, either directly or through an insurance broker. A sales representative from the HMO (or the broker) meets with the employer to learn about his or her business and coverage needs, and to present information about the HMO and its benefit plans.

If the employer finds the HMO and its benefits attractive, the employer selects one particular benefit plan to cover all its employees, and then asks for a quote. The HMO representative works with the employer to prepare a list of employees called an *employee census.* The employee census includes basic demographic information for each employee, such as age, sex and number of dependents.

The census is sent to the HMO for analysis. Using the information provided in the census, certain characteristics of the employer's business and the benefit plan selected, the HMO's Underwriting department determines the premium rates for the group (for a description of this process, see Rating and Underwriting on page 83.) These rates are presented to the employer as a formal quote which is guaranteed for thirty days. When the employer accepts the quoted rates, a contract is signed by both parties. The HMO then works with the employer to enroll the employees of the new group.

The Open Enrollment Period

People with employer-sponsored health coverage can join HMOs in one of two ways. New employees and their families may join an HMO at the point they become eligible for health benefits. Established employees may change their health plans during an *open enrollment period.*

Open enrollment is a period of time, usually one month per year, during which employees and their dependents may move from one health coverage option to another without any special requirements or restrictions. Also, dependents who may not have been covered under the employer's plan for some reason may be added at this time. In some nonqualified plans, people desiring to move into an alternate plan outside of the open enrollment period may be required to complete a medical questionnaire or submit to a medical examination in order to obtain coverage (for a discussion, please see page 82.)

Eligibility Requirements

Eligibility requirements for HMO coverage are established through a combination of HMO and employer policies.

Requirements established by the employer may include completion of a probationary period or working a minimum number of hours per week to qualify for benefits. Policies commonly set by the HMO include requirements that enrollees must live or work in the HMO's service area, the subscriber must be a *bona fide* employee (active or retired) of the employer group, and covered family members must be legal dependents of the subscriber.

A particularly important requirement centers on the member's selection of a primary care physician. Most HMOs now allow individuals in the same family to choose different PCPs from within the same medical group. For instance, a woman might choose an internist, while her husband has a family practitioner and the kids see a pediatrician. Some plans may allow a woman to choose a gynecologist as her PCP. Additionally, many IPA and network HMOs permit families to select their PCPs from among physicians in different medical groups. Some health plans still require that the subscriber choose one PCP for the whole family, but this is becoming less common. In such cases, all family members must receive care from the same PCP and medical group.

Dependents are covered by most HMOs through 18 years of age – this is known as the *dependent cutoff age*. The cutoff age may extend through 23 years of age for full time students, but this age can vary according to the needs of the employer group. When enrolling a full-time student dependent, keep in mind that if the student's college residence is not within the service area of the HMO, the student may be covered only for emergencies when away at school. This is because routine care must be received from contracting providers, and an HMO does not contract with providers outside of its service area. Usually, students are covered for routine care only if they return to the service area. Some plans now offer *student riders* for an additional premium. Through the rider, the student has indemnity-style health coverage while away at school and can use the HMO coverage when at home. Also, some multi-state HMOs have reciprocity arrangements that allow subsidiaries in one state to coordinate cover age with their out-of-state affiliates.

New dependents typically must be enrolled within 30 days of becoming eligible for coverage – new spouses within 30 days of marriage, newborns within 30 days of birth, and newly-adopted children within 30 days of placement. Young families should find out how their HMO extends coverage to newborns. Some states require that HMOs cover a new baby for the first 30 days after birth, even if the baby is not subsequently enrolled in the plan. In other states, HMOs provide coverage only if the baby is enrolled within 30 days and premiums are paid retroactive to the date of birth. Most HMOs are very good about reminding new parents to enroll their newborn within the time limit, but the financial consequences of not doing so can be considerable – it pays to be informed.

The Enrollment Process

After the employer signs the HMO enrollment contract, its employees are given the opportunity to enroll in the HMO through an open enrollment period. Each employee selecting the plan completes an application with personal and dependent information. The employees' applications are then sent to the HMO along with the group's premium.

Community Health Plan				
Name _____ Sex _____				
DOB _____ ID Number _____				
Primary Physician _____				
24-Hour Telephone _____				
Benefit	OV	Hosp	RX	MH	ER
Copay	$5	$100	$7	$25	$25

Figure 3. Sample HMO Identification Card

Upon receipt by the HMO, information from the applications is entered into the plan's computer system. Each new member is linked with the employer's selected benefit plan and the member's chosen PCP. Once enrolled, the employee is called the *subscriber;* the subscriber and dependents are all referred to as *enrollees* or *members* of the HMO. Coverage normally begins on the first day of the month specified by the employer.

Most HMOs provide their members with *membership cards* or *ID cards* which members use to identify themselves to plan providers. In some HMOs, one card is issued to the subscriber for the whole family; more commonly, plans issue a separate ID card for each enrollee. Figure 3 presents one popular card format that includes copayment information. After entering the new members' data into its computer system, the HMO mails ID cards to the new members, along with enrollment materials that explain the HMO's policies and procedures. These materials vary by HMO, but usually consist of the following documents.

❏ A document called a *Summary Plan Description, Evidence of Coverage* or *Coverage Certificate* summarizes the main provisions of the group contract through which the member is enrolled. The Summary includes lists of covered benefits and benefit limitations; required copayment or coinsurance amounts; services and types of care that are excluded from coverage; and eligibility and enrollment policies.

❏ A *Disclosure Form* explains how to obtain services through the HMO, procedures for obtaining emergency care inside and outside the service area, and for changing primary care physicians. Also included are descriptions of the service area and the HMO's lock-in requirement; the procedures for obtaining authorizations and referrals; coordination of benefits policies; and grievance and appeals procedures. Alternatively, this information may be included in the Summary Plan Description.

❏ A *Provider Directory* describes the HMO's provider network – its primary care physicians and physician groups, with their locations and telephone numbers; participating hospitals and pharmacies in the plan's service area; and the names of specialist physicians available on referral through plan PCPs.

Retroactivity and Enrollment

Retroactivity is a term used to describe situations in which the prepaid basis for HMO care must be adjusted to account for the timing of prior events. It is an accounting concept that is useful for reconciling premium and capitation payments, should the HMO's records of member effective dates differ from those of the employer or medical group.

Retroactivity is an issue that the HMO member seldom sees, and is presented here only so that the reader has an idea of the complexities involved in administering prepaid care. Retroactivity can be best understood with an example:

February 11th. Betty Thomas signs up for the Presto HMO, expecting to be covered beginning on **March 1st.** She turns in her enrollment forms to the personnel office at work and makes an appointment to see her new PCP.

March 15th. At her doctor appointment, she tells the receptionist that she's just joined the HMO and doesn't have an ID card yet, but the receptionist doesn't call the HMO to verify eligibility. The doctor gives her a physical and tells her everything seems fine.

March 17th. Back at her work, Betty's enrollment form is discovered at the bottom of a mail bag. The mail clerk dutifully recovers it and sends it on to the Presto HMO.

March 21st. Betty's enrollment application is processed, and the HMO makes her coverage effective on **April 1st.** The HMO mails her an ID card and enrollment packet.

March 25th. She receives her HMO enrollment materials. She puts the ID card in her purse and the enrollment materials wind up in a drawer. She doesn't read them.

April 2nd. Betty receives a bill from her PCP with a note that the bill had been denied by the medical group because she was not a Presto HMO member on the date of her examination. She contacts the personnel office at work to find out what went wrong.

April 3rd. The personnel manager explains the problem to the HMO. The HMO realizes that a mistake was made and makes her coverage retroactive to **March 1st.**

April 4th. Presto HMO staff prepare a statement to bill Betty's employer for one month of retroactive premium; this corrects the employer's account. The HMO also adjusts the medical group's capitation for one additional month of retroactivity; this corrects the medical group account. The medical group then can pay the PCP for the March 15th visit, and the world is back in synch.

In the example, the member and her employer believed that she was covered as of March 1st; the HMO and medical group records, however, showed her with coverage effective April 1st, and were out of synch with those of the member and employer. The retroactive transactions – one for billing and one for capitation – effectively resynchronized the records of the various parties.

Obviously, one small event can create a retroactivity situation that requires some work to resolve. Most HMO enrollees will never experience a retroactivity problem like the one illustrated in the example. However, it is useful to be acquainted with the concept of retroactivity should such a situation ever arise.

•

Once enrolled, most HMO members simply begin to receive care through their chosen PCP as needed, with little further interaction with the HMO. Aside from occasional communications from the HMO – a member newsletter, for example – the HMO works unobtrusively behind the scenes to administer the health care of its members.

5. Managing Care in HMOs

This chapter discusses the major methods used by HMOs to manage the quality and cost of health services provided to HMO members. These methods work together to accomplish several objectives: they reduce the frequency of unnecessary services, assure that services are provided in the most appropriate setting, and promote the use of contracting providers to maintain the quality and cost effectiveness of care.

Referrals and Authorizations

The primary care physician is expected to provide all routine care that a patient may need, and to evaluate the need for secondary and acute care services of specialists, therapists and hospitals. When an HMO patient needs specialist care, the PCP sends the patient to a specialist through a *referral.*

In IPA and network plans, the "arm's length" relationship between the HMO and the medical group results in a formal referral process based on written requests. In most cases, the specialist belongs to the PCP's medical group or participates in the HMO's provider network. The PCP records the referral on a special *referral form* that provides clinical information on the patient and documents that the patient was referred by the PCP. The form is sent to the specialist along with the patient or by mail.

The patient then makes an appointment with the specialist. In consultation, the specialist evaluates the patient for the problem described in the referral and may perform diagnostic tests and procedures if needed. After seeing the patient, the specialist uses the referral form to report back to the PCP about the patient's condition, and to bill the medical group or HMO for services.

In many group and and staff-model HMOs, the referral process is relatively informal – the patient is simply directed to make an appointment to see the specialist at the next available appointment. A referral form may be used to convey clinical information, but has no role in billing.

In many HMOs, especially network and IPA-model plans, the patient's physician must obtain *authorization* from the HMO or the medical group before complex secondary or acute care services can be provided. In urgent cases, requests for authorization may be telephoned or sent by fax machine; routine requests are often mailed. Based on the information provided by the requesting physician, a medical director or utilization reviewer evaluates the patient's symptoms, the appropriateness of the proposed treatment or procedure, and possible alternatives. Once approved, an authorization is issued; in most cases, requests can be processed within 24 to 48 hours of receipt.

In staff and group-model plans, we have noted that physicians are more integrated into the HMO's operations and administration, and that more services are provided in-house. As a result, authorizations and referrals have less importance, except when services are to be furnished through "outside" providers under contract. The following example illustrates how the authorization and referral systems might function in a typical IPA or network setting:

> An HMO member has been having crampy stomach pain off and on for several weeks. The patient consults his PCP who believes that the symptoms may indicate the presence of gallstones. However, the PCP feels that a specialist's opinion is needed in order to be certain.

The PCP completes a referral form to refer the patient to a participating IPA surgeon for evaluation. One copy of the referral is given to the patient and another is sent to the IPA. (note that the PCP's referral to the specialist is at the PCP's discretion – since the specialist is part of the PCP's IPA, no formal review or approval is required.)

The patient makes an appointment to see the specialist the following week. On examination, the surgeon suspects that the patient has gallstones, but needs to confirm the diagnosis through an ultrasound examination. The IPA is financially responsible for this service under its contract with the HMO, so he contacts the IPA medical director to request approval of the ultrasound. The surgeon receives approval the next day. He completes a second referral form for the patient and arranges to have the exam done the next day in the radiology department of a contracting hospital.

When the patient's ultrasound exam is completed, the test results are sent to the specialist, who contacts the PCP the next day and informs her that the diagnosis is confirmed. In this case, he says, surgical removal of the gallbladder is the preferred treatment.

The surgeon proposes to perform the operation using a technique called 'laparoscopic cholecystectomy' in which the gall bladder is removed using a special viewing scope inserted into the patient's abdomen through the skin. The procedure requires only a small incision with local anesthesia, and can be performed in an ambulatory surgery clinic. The laparoscopic procedure causes the patient much less discomfort and has fewer complications than conventional gall bladder surgery.

The PCP agrees with the specialist's recommendations and gives her consent to the procedure. The specialist then contacts the HMO's Authorization department to obtain authorization. By telephone, he explains his findings, the rationale for treatment and the proposed procedure. The request is reviewed by an HMO medical director or nurse reviewer who considers the following:

- Is the treatment medically necessary?
- Is the treatment the most appropriate for the patient's condition?
- Will the procedure be performed in the most appropriate setting?
- Is the specialist qualified to perform the procedure?
- Is the patient currently a member of the HMO with coverage for the proposed procedure?

If the medical director or reviewer is satisfied that the criteria are met, he or she approves the procedure. A written authorization is prepared and copies sent to the specialist, the IPA and the hospital where the procedure will take place. The specialist may then proceed to make arrangements to perform the procedure.

In a small percentage of requests, authorization is denied because the HMO or medical group decides that the procedure is not medically necessary or is inappropriate for the patient's condition. In such cases, the medical director will deny the request and the service will not be covered. This does not mean that the patient cannot receive the service or procedure – only that the HMO will not pay for it.

The medical director may work with the requesting physician, suggesting alternate therapies or treatment settings that are more appropriate to the patient's situation. If the member believes that the HMO is denying coverage of the service unfairly, he or she may appeal the denials through the HMO's Grievance and Appeals System (please see Chapter 9.)

Referral and authorization systems are designed to control utilization by preventing self-referral and decreasing the number of unnecessary procedures. It is worth noting that the mere presence of an authorization or referral system can have a "watch-dog" effect, and is often enough to deter providers from performing unnecessary procedures.

Authorization and referral requirements are an aspect of HMO membership that some people have difficulty with at first. As an HMO member, there are several important points to remember about authorizations and referrals that will help you to deal with them more easily:

- HMOs require authorizations and referrals for many non-routine services – make sure you know when they apply. These policies should be explained in your Summary Plan Description, but ask your PCP about anything that is unclear.

- Be actively involved in your care – ask your physician if he or she has obtained the necessary approvals before you have a procedure done.

- Most authorizations and referrals are given for specific services from a specific provider. You must obtain services only from the authorized provider, and the provider cannot provide additional services without additional authorization.

- Some kinds of authorized or referral services must be performed within a certain time period. Ask if your referral has an expiration date – if so, make sure your appointment is scheduled before then, particularly in the case of specialists.

- Ongoing authorizations are sometimes given for services related to chronic or long term conditions, but the HMO may require periodic reviews to determine that services are still necessary.

Utilization Review

HMOs can provide quality care for less money because their utilization management systems are effective in controlling unnecessary utilization, and this reduces costs. Some of these systems control utilization before it occurs, as with primary care physician gatekeepers and authorization systems. *Utilization review (UR)* – also called *concurrent review* – is different in that services are monitored as they are provided.

The majority of utilization review programs center on inpatient services, such as acute hospitalization, because these services are the most expensive. UR staff from the HMO are composed of nurses and physicians who work with hospital UR staff to monitor care being provided to the HMO's members.

Utilization review works like this: at regular intervals, UR staff from the HMO assess the progress of each of the HMO's hospitalized members through reviews of medical records and interviews with attending physicians and hospital staff. In many plans, reviewers visit each hospital where HMO patients are admitted – this is called *on-site review.* When distance makes on-site review impractical, information may be obtained through *telephonic review* – a combination of telephone conversation and facsimile transmissions. Some patients may be reviewed on a daily basis if their condition requires it, while more stable patients are reviewed every few days.

Through its UR system, the HMO continuously gathers current information on the clinical status of each of its hospitalized members. The reviewers evaluate each case according to basic utilization criteria, such as:

• Is the setting (ICU, surgical ward, etc.) appropriate to the patient's condition?

• Is hospitalization still necessary?

• Is the patient receiving appropriate and effective treatment?

Utilization review provides several significant advantages. The attending physician gains additional clinical resources in the form of the HMO medical director and data from the HMO's quality management and technology assessment programs. With ongoing review, the HMO knows when the patient is ready for discharge, and can coordinate with the attending physician so that the patient doesn't remain in the hospital any longer than necessary.

Furthermore, utilization review promotes conformance to the HMO's standards of care (see page 105.) With a UR system in place, physicians are less likely to practice in a vacuum or outside of the mainstream of care. Through medical directors and reviewers, the HMO can involve itself in the clinical decisions affecting its enrollees and can ensure that its standards of care are maintained through ongoing discussions with the attending physicians.

Alternatives to Hospitalization

Most people are admitted to hospitals because they need the specialized intensive 24-hour care that only a hospital can provide. Historically, though, many patients have been admitted because they needed diagnostic tests or surgical procedures that were available only through the hospital. Also, it has not been uncommon for people to be admitted as a matter of convenience for them or their physicians.

Increasing costs and advances in medical technology over the past twenty years years have played a large part in changing the rationale for admitting a patient to the hospital. In particular, progress in diagnostic electronics and imaging, and the availability of new anesthetics and drugs that are less toxic to the patient have meant that the traditional role of the hospital has changed considerably.

Definitive care for many conditions can now be safely provided in non-hospital settings, and HMOs have consistently been in the forefront in integrating these alternatives to hospitalization into their provider networks, authorization criteria and standards of care. In many cases, treatment in alternative settings results in lower costs, less inconvenience for the patient, and reduced incidence of complications. The following are some alternatives that have found broad acceptance in HMOs:

❏ **Alternative birthing centers (ABCs)** are special facilities where women can deliver babies in a home-like environment using natural childbirth techniques. As a result of physicians' greater confidence in identifying uncomplicated pregnancies, the increased use of nurse-midwives, and the trend away from the routine use of anesthetics, ABCs have gained increased acceptance as a safe, low-cost alternative to a hospital delivery.

❏ **Home IV (intravenous) therapy** has been made practical through electronically-controlled pumps and infusion devices, and through significant advances in pharmacology and biochemistry.

❏ **Ambulatory surgery units** have shifted a great number of patients from hospital beds to outpatient settings. For years, the principle danger of surgery has been the side effects of anesthesia, not the operation itself. New short-acting anesthetics are much safer for patients, resulting in fewer complications. Combined with new less-invasive surgical techniques and technology such as fiberoptic scopes and lasers, many patients can undergo a surgical procedure without being admitted to the hospital, and leave soon after the procedure to recover at home.

❏ **Diagnostic testing** has been changed significantly by advances in fields such as magnetic resonance imaging (MRI) and CAT scans, ultrasound, nuclear medicine and laboratory automation. Combined with the realization that many tests can be done safely and reliably on an outpatient basis, the old notion of being "admitted for a few tests" has practically vanished – it is simply no longer cost-effective. Accordingly, HMOs require that most diagnostic testing be done in an outpatient setting prior to admission.

❏ **Home health care** permits many patients to be discharged from the hospital sooner in order to recover from an illness at home. HMOs provide a variety of services in the home, including skilled nursing, rehabilitation therapy services and home IV therapy. There are several advantages to the home care approach. The patient can recover in familiar, safer and more-comfortable surroundings. Also, care provided at home is often less expensive than care given in a hospital or other facility.

Case Management

Case management is a process of working with the various providers involved in a patient's care to monitor the patient's condition and catch problems before they become serious. HMOs use case management to coordinate and monitor the care provided to patients with complex medical problems. It often begins before discharge from the hospital and continues through convalescence. Patients with complex long-term problems may receive case management services on an ongoing basis for years. In some plans, case managers may have "specialties" – coordinating out-of-area cases, managing high-risk pregnancies or serving patients with multiple disabilities. The goals of case management are straightforward:

- Return the patient to the level of functioning and activity he or she had prior to the illness

- Monitor the patient for signs of complications or other problems so early treatment can be started

- Ensure that the post-discharge care provided by various practitioners is coordinated and effective, and to facilitate communication among those involved

Case management is accomplished through *case conferences* with care providers. Several times each week, a case manager reviews the patient's progress with each of the providers involved in the patient's care, e.g. home care nurses, IV therapy nurses, physical therapists and social workers. The case manager is then in a position to combine the clinical information received from these care providers and present a complete picture of the patient's progress to the attending physician.

If a problem or warning sign is noted, the patient's physician can be notified quickly and the appropriate treatment started. Rarely, this may mean readmission to the hospital; most of the time, though, a simple diagnostic test, change in medication or minor procedure is enough to correct the problem, and readmission to the hospital is avoided.

Case management programs are now coming into use outside of HMOs as insurance companies realize their effectiveness. For years, they have been a standard component of HMO operations because they get results. Case management complements and supports the physician's coordination of patient care. It works in the interest of the patient because of its emphasis on prevention and rehabilitation, and in the HMO's interest because it promotes quality and helps manage costs.

Generic Drugs and Formularies

When a new drug first enters the market, the drug company that owns the drug patent has exclusive rights to make and market the drug for a number of years. In this initial period, the company markets the drug under its brand name and tries to maximize sales of the drug to recover its investment and make a profit. When the period of exclusivity comes to an end, other drug companies may begin to produce non-brand versions of the drug; these are known as *generic drugs.*

Generics are chemically identical to the original drugs, but may contain different inactive ingredients or be made by different methods. In nearly all cases, the medical profession considers generics to be as safe and effective as their brand-name counterparts. Also, generics cost less than brand-name drugs. They are so widely accepted that over two-thirds of American HMOs have instituted *mandatory generic programs.* These programs require that generic drugs be dispensed to enrollees instead of a brand-name, when an acceptable generic equivalent is available.

A *drug formulary* is a list containing the names of certain prescription drugs that an HMO covers when dispensed to its members who have drug coverage. Developing a formulary requires a significant amount of research, analysis of options, and consensus building among HMO physicians. As an alternative, an HMO may acquire a commercially-developed formulary program and implement it with the cooperation of the HMO's contracting medical groups and physicians. Once in place, the formulary must be reviewed and updated regularly to remain current with new developments in pharmacology and medical practice.

Whether developed by the HMO's physicians or by a consultant, a well-designed formulary can accomplish several objectives. Formularies can enhance the overall quality of care because they can be structured to include only those drugs that are most widely used in modern medical practice, and exclude those that are marginally effective, overly expensive, or have become obsolete.

Formularies can serve as vehicles for implementing mandatory generic programs. A formulary can be designed to identify the acceptable generic equivalents of brand-name drugs and the situations where brand-name drugs may be covered. Finally, formularies promote cost-effectiveness by steering physicians and pharmacists toward the most effective drugs in their most appropriate and cost-effective forms.

•

The utilization management systems described in this chapter work together to minimize provision of unnecessary medical services and to involve the HMO in the patient's care. These systems represent the most direct interaction between the HMO and its contracted providers in the course of providing care to HMO members. While they are significant in controlling costs, their greatest importance lies in the fact that they permit the HMO to influence the quality of care provided and the ultimate outcome of the patient's treatment.

6. HMO Benefits and Plan Design

Most health maintenance organizations offer a range of *benefit plans,* which are distinct combinations of certain characteristics, such as limitations, copayments, optional benefits, rating methods and premiums. Benefit plans range from deluxe designs with low copayments and enhanced coverage to no-frills plans with basic coverage and higher copayments. With a variety of benefit plans, HMOs try to satisfy the varying needs of different employer groups. When an employer signs a coverage contract with an HMO, the employer essentially selects one particular benefit plan to cover all of its employees, even though that benefit plan may consist of several options.

Benefit Structure

Federally-qualified HMOs – those which meet the federal government's basic HMO requirements – must offer a minimum set of covered benefits in each of their benefit plans*. Also known as *mandated benefits,* these minimum benefits serve as a benchmark for the HMO industry as a whole. For this reason, we will use them as a model for discussing benefits in the typical HMO.

There are two kinds of mandated benefits. *Basic benefits* must be provided to all HMO members as standard components of coverage. *Supplemental benefits* are benefits that an HMO must make available, either as standard benefits

---

* Federally-qualified HMOs may establish certain "non-qualified" product lines in addition to their federally-qualified products. Non-qualified products may or may not conform to federal qualification regulations.
For more information on mandated benefits, see *Code of Federal Regulations, Title 42, Chapter 4, Section 417.101.*

or through a *rider* – an optional coverage enhancement which provides additional benefits at extra cost. Basic mandated benefits include the following:

- Physician services
- Outpatient diagnostic and treatment services
- Inpatient hospital services
- Short-term rehabilitation and physical therapy
- Mental health outpatient visits, up to twenty per year
- Emergencies in and out of the HMO's service area
- Detoxification and treatment of substance abuse
- Diagnostic laboratory services
- Diagnostic and therapeutic radiology services
- Home health services
- Preventive health services, including the following:
  - family planning services
  - infertility diagnosis and treatment
  - well-child care
  - periodic health exams (annual physicals)
  - eye and ear exams for children through age 17
  - pediatric and adult immunizations

Designating certain services as basic benefits creates several advantages for HMO members. With few exceptions, HMOs cannot limit basic benefit services to a maximum number of services or a maximum dollar benefit. HMO enrollees are assured that they will receive basic benefits whenever necessary. Also, through basic benefits, HMOs makes it easy for enrollees to obtain preventive care.

In federally-qualified HMOs, the distinction between basic and supplemental benefits is also significant because of a federal requirement that sets annual *out-of-pocket limits* on the total amount of copayments that can be required of an HMO enrollee. Under this provision, total annual copayments made for basic benefit services cannot exceed 200% of the total annual premiums which would be charged for a comparable HMO benefit plan *with no copayments.*

Many HMOs calculate their annual out-of-pocket limit once each year, and then publish the limit amount in their member newsletter. Members must keep track of copayments and notify the HMO when this annual limit is reached. At that point, the member's obligation to make copayments for basic services ends until the following calendar year. Since copayments made for supplemental services do not count toward the annual limit, most people never come close to reaching the annual limit. However, this provision can be of real value to people covered under benefit plans with hospital copayments who are admitted to the hospital several times during a year.

Supplemental benefits can consist of any services that are not included in the list of basic benefits. Federal HMO regulations describe a number of specific services which HMOs may offer, but aren't required to provide. However, many HMOs choose to offer one or more of these services as basic benefits. Common examples would be inclusion of vision care or blood products under standard coverage.

Other supplemental benefits, such as durable medical equipment, prescription drugs, dental care and optical services, usually are offered as riders that employer groups may select as options. HMOs may place limits on these services in forms such as a yearly maximum number of visits or a maximum dollar benefit per member.

Limitations and Exclusions

Limitations are restrictions placed on a benefit to either: 1) restrict the circumstances under which a benefit can be used; or 2) place a ceiling on the number of services or the total value of services covered under a benefit. *Exclusions* are services or procedures which are not covered benefits under any circumstances. Limitations and exclusions are a part of any health coverage policy, whether through an indemnity carrier or an HMO. While the two concepts are straightforward, they deserve mention because they are often misunderstood by enrollees and may not be well-explained in plan materials.

Some HMOs have benefit limitations and exclusions which vary by benefit plan. However, for ease of administration, many HMOs develop a single set of limitations and exclusions which are then used in all benefit plan designs. They are typically explained in the Summary Plan Description immediately following the Benefits section.

Limitations

Most limitations are established for supplemental benefits. They may also affect basic benefits to the extent permitted by federal qualification regulations:

- **Skilled nursing facility** care is commonly limited to 30, 60 or 100 days per calendar year

- **Eyeglasses and corrective lenses** are provided only once every year or two (usually as a rider)

- **Mental health inpatient services** are often restricted to 30 days per year

- Coverage of **blood** may be limited to units which are subsequently replaced through a blood bank donation

Exclusions

HMO exclusions are similar to the exclusions used by traditional indemnity insurers. Some exclusions result from an underlying view that medical coverage should not include care for conditions which are not essentially related to health or illness. Others seem to derive from the *allopathic model* of medicine predominant in the United States. The allopathic model of medicine is based on treating disease through the identification and treatment of physical signs and symptoms. This model effectively determines what is accepted within the scope of medical practice and, therefore, what is covered by medical insurance. The following are typical exclusions:

- **Custodial or convalescent care** – does not require the services of medical professionals

- **Cosmetic surgery** – cosmetic procedures are not essentially related to health or illness

- **Dental care** – not within the scope of medical care, but sometimes offered as a rider

- **Chiropractic, acupuncture and other alternative therapies** – also considered outside the scope of medical care, but sometimes sold in riders

- **Experimental procedures** – these are procedures which are not yet integrated into accepted medical practice and are of unproven effectiveness

- **Routine foot care** – not essentially medical in nature; can be performed by unlicensed personnel

- **Services which are work-related** – excluded because laws of most states make worker's compensation insurance responsible for covering occupational illnesses and injuries

- **Obesity treatment** – considered to be a behavioral rather than medical problem, despite the link between obesity and the development of cardiac and other systemic disease; diets and psychological treatments are open-ended and expensive

- **Sex change operations** – not considered medically necessary

- **High-tech infertility procedures** such as *in vitro* fertilization and zygote intrafallopian transfer *(ZIFT)*

Prescription Drug Benefits

Prescription drug coverage is so widely offered through riders by HMOs that it deserves a special mention. While medications in the hospital and injectable medications administered to an outpatient by a physician or nurse are covered as basic benefits, prescription drug riders provide coverage for outpatient prescription medicines that the patient can self-administer. Copayments are quite common, ranging from $2 to $15 per prescription; most plans charge one copayment for each 30-day supply. In nearly all cases, over-the-counter drugs and supplies are not covered.

To further control prescription drug expenses, about two-thirds of HMOs use formularies, and more than two-thirds have mandatory generic programs. In such a program, the HMO requires that the generic form of a drug be dispensed if an accepted generic is available. As an alternative, some HMOs have adopted *tiered copayment* structures to encourage members to use generic drugs. When a member requests a brand-name drug, he or she pays a higher copayment; when the generic equivalent is dispensed, there is a lower copayment. The average generic copayment is about $5 versus $7 when a brand-name drug is dispensed.

The amount of a prescription drug that may be dispensed at any one time is restricted in many HMOs. Some HMOs limit the quantity dispensed to a 30 or 60-day supply because many drugs require monitoring by a physician to watch for possible side effects. Also, HMOs are understandably reluctant to issue several month's supply of a medication to someone who could terminate his or her HMO membership in the following month.

Staff and group model plans often operate pharmacies in their outpatient facilities – this approach is convenient to patients, a useful resource for physicians, and cost-effective for the HMO. Many large IPA and network-model HMOs administer their prescription drug benefits through large prescription service networks. These networks provide chain drug stores and many independent pharmacies with computerized eligibility and coverage information, and prescription claims processing for HMO enrollees. To further increase convenience and reduce costs, some HMOs encourage members to use mail-order prescription drug services, especially those members with ongoing medication needs.

Other Forms of HMO Coverage

As we have seen, HMOs typically incorporate certain managed-care techniques into their operations: utilization controls, prepaid reimbursement, contracted provider networks, primary care physician gatekeepers, etc. In some cases, though, HMOs have had to depart from these classic managed-care methods to be responsive to the needs of the health care market, and remain competitive with other forms of health insurance coverage.

Employers wishing to offer HMO coverage may face several common problems in setting up benefit plans that meet the needs of all their employees. These problems include employee resistance to the unfamiliar concepts of "HMOs" and "managed care"; workers who may not live within the service area of an HMO; and employees who want to see a doctor who isn't an HMO network provider. In response, many HMOs develop alternatives to their standard HMO plans. Some of these alternatives offer more flexibility in provider selection because they incorporate elements of PPO and indemnity coverage.

❑ *Multiple Option Plans (MOPs)* allow the employee a choice of two or more coverage options – such as HMO, PPO or indemnity – through the same health plan. At the time of enrollment, the employee chooses one plan option for his or her entire family, and they remain covered under the chosen option until the next annual open enrollment period. If the family resides in the HMO service area, they can choose any of the options; if outside the HMO service area, the family can still be covered by indemnity or through the PPO. If they become dissatisfied with their choice, they can switch to another coverage option during the next open enrollment.

Financial incentives in these plans encourage enrollees to select care through the less-expensive HMO option. Although care must be obtained from participating HMO providers, enrollees in the HMO option enjoy higher levels of benefits, lower copayments and no deductibles.

Coverage through the PPO or indemnity options is available to those willing to pay more for a wider choice of providers. The trade-offs under these options are higher premiums, lower levels of benefits, coinsurance instead of copayments, and annual deductibles.

❏ *Point of Service (POS)* products allow the enrollee to choose HMO, PPO or indemnity coverage at the point of service, i.e., at the time services are received. Some POS plans have only two coverage options available (HMO and indemnity); these are sometimes called *opt-out* or *swing-out* plans. As with MOPs, financial incentives encourage the enrollee to receive care from providers in the HMO network. Services received on a PPO or indemnity basis are still covered, but are subject to higher copayments, coinsurance and/or deductibles; benefits also may be reduced.

Unlike MOPs, POS products allow people to try managed care without having to make a one-year commitment. Enrollees may choose to receive care outside the network at any time, so utilization controls are not as effective in reducing costs of care in POS plans. Therefore, premiums are higher than for regular HMO coverage.

Like MOPs, POS plans are also attractive to employers whose employees are located over a wide geographic area. Even though some employees may be located outside the HMO's service area, they may be able to receive care and coverage under the PPO or indemnity components of the POS plan.

Many states do not permit HMOs to pay directly for expenses incurred on an indemnity or PPO basis. As a result, in many POS products, claims for members under the indemnity and PPO segments are paid by an indemnity insurer working with the HMO in a joint venture.

❏ *Self-Funded HMO.* Self-funded HMOs combine an HMO and its network with an employer who directly underwrites the cost of medical care for its employees. Employees receive care from the same providers as regular HMO enrollees, but their care is paid for with the employer's funds, rather than funds from the HMO. The employer contracts with the HMO for access to its provider network, and may purchase other services, such as utilization management and claims processing.

Continuation of Coverage

While the majority of HMO members receive their coverage through a commercial employer group, individuals can continue their HMO benefits even if they lose coverage through their employer. Several forms of coverage are available for such individuals.

COBRA coverage is one method of continuing benefits which applies to all types of health coverage. COBRA health care laws are part of federal legislation called the *Consolidated Omnibus Budget Reconciliation Act of 1985.* COBRA coverage is available to people who would otherwise lose their coverage due to circumstances such as a layoff, reduction in hours, death of spouse, Medicare eligibility, divorce, employer bankruptcy or job change.

If an employer is subject to COBRA (for example, a business with 20 or more employees), an individual employee or dependent who would otherwise lose his or her health coverage can maintain the same level of benefits at the same premium offered to the employer for a period of up to 18 or 36 months, depending on the circumstances. The individual makes premium payments directly to the employer for the duration of the COBRA period, and may have to pay an administrative fee of up to two percent. The employer then maintains the individual's coverage in the HMO. Employees who are terminated for gross misconduct are not eligible for COBRA coverage.

Conversion plans are another means of continuing coverage. They are offered by most HMOs to members who lose their employer-based benefits. These plans are designed to provide coverage for individuals whose COBRA coverage has expired; for dependent adult children who lose their full-time student status; or in cases where the employer is exempt from COBRA. Unlike COBRA, most conversion plans offer fewer benefits at a higher premium. Still, they offer a means for maintaining coverage in the HMO until other employer-based coverage can be obtained.

Many traditional insurance companies don't offer conversion plans. Most HMOs do offer conversion, so this is yet another advantage of HMOs. Make sure the HMO you join offers conversion, especially if you think you might need it someday. Eligibility requirements for COBRA and conversion plans are quite complex and subject to legal restrictions. Should you ever need to continue your coverage through such a plan, be sure to discuss your specific situation with your benefits administrator or HMO.

Medicare Coverage and HMOs

HMOs can cover people with Medicare in one of several ways - through *Medicare supplement* plans or through plans based on contracts with Medicare (known as *Medicare risk* and *Medicare cost contracts).* Most HMOs offer retiree coverage either through employer-sponsored retirement packages or on an individual basis. In this section, we examine HMO/ Medicare coverage and Medicare's rules for those who continue to work after age 65.

Medicare and the "Working Aged" Rules

Increasingly, people are choosing to continue to work after reaching age 65. People with Medicare who continue to work are subject to special rules, and it is important to understand how the rules relate to other health coverage.

Medicare consists of two parts: *Part A* (hospital insurance) and *Part B* (medical insurance for physician and other services.) Most people become entitled to Medicare upon reaching age 65 or by becoming permanently disabled. The majority of those with Medicare receive Part A at no cost, but Part B is available only by paying a premium to Medicare. As a result, most people don't apply for Part B until after they retire.

If an individual with Medicare also has health coverage through an employer, Medicare requires that the employer-based coverage pays first (the *primary payer*) and Medicare pays for any remaining amounts (the *secondary payer*). Medicare's policy is presented in a complex set of rules called the *working aged* or *secondary payer* rules. The rules are summarized here to give you an idea of when Medicare would be secondary to your HMO coverage.

If you are 65 or over and have Medicare coverage, and you or your spouse continues to work, and the employer provides group health coverage, then the working aged rules apply:

1) If the employer has 20 or more employees, you may:

   • keep the group health coverage and Medicare will pay secondary to the group coverage; or

   • reject the group health coverage and Medicare will pay as primary payer; in this case, the employer may not pay for any Medicare supplement.

2) If the employer has fewer than 20 employees, Medicare will pay as the primary payer.

Other circumstances in which Medicare is the secondary payer include:

- for work-related illnesses and injuries covered by worker's compensation

- coverage for certain disabled persons who are covered through their employer or spouse

The law requires that employers offer employees and spouses who are 65 and older the same coverage offered to younger employees and spouses. The employer cannot deny you coverage or offer a different or reduced set of benefits because you have Medicare. For more information on the secondary payer rules and how they apply in specific cases, contact your employer's benefits administrator or your local Social Security Administration office.

Medicare Supplements

In *Medicare supplement plans,* Medicare continues to be the member's primary insurer. The HMO's coverage "wraps around" the benefits provided through Medicare, covering some or all of the deductibles and coinsurance that Medicare beneficiaries must normally pay. With supplements, the member is not "locked in" to the HMO provider network in the normal sense. The member may receive care from non-network providers and Medicare will pay for it; however, the HMO may not cover claims from non-network providers.

To receive coverage through the HMO, the member must obtain care through HMO network providers and follow the HMO's referral and authorization requirements when applicable. Out-of-pocket costs for the enrollee can be lower than with regular Medicare, depending on the proportion of services received through the HMO. Individual supplement plans cost somewhat more than regular HMO commercial coverage, and may be priced much higher than Medicare contract plans.

Medicare Contract Plans

Medicare contract plans work quite differently and are much less expensive than supplements. These plans are available to individual and group retirees through HMOs that contract with the Medicare program (HCFA) to provide managed care to Medicare members. There are two types: *Medicare cost HMOs* are paid by HCFA based on the costs of the care they provide, while *Medicare risk HMOs* are paid on a prepaid capitation basis. Medicare risk HMOs have clearly emerged as the more popular of the two, so we will focus only on Medicare risk HMOs in this section.

In a Medicare risk plan, the member must receive all of his or her Medicare benefits through the HMO. The HMO then administers those benefits, provides the member with all services normally covered through Medicare, and covers the annual deductibles and coinsurance as well. Risk plans may offer benefits not usually covered by Medicare; in group retiree plans, the employer also may pay for further benefit enhancements, such as prescription drug coverage. In either kind of plan, all claims are paid through the HMO; if claims are sent to Medicare, Medicare will reject them because its records show that the member is assigned to a contracting Medicare risk HMO.

Should the member decide to withdraw from a Medicare plan, he or she may do so by contacting the plan or through a Social Security office. Disenrollments are usually effective the first of the month following the disenrollment request, and the member is reinstated into regular fee-for-service Medicare.

Medicare risk HMOs take their name from the fact that the HMO assumes all financial risk and responsibility for providing the member with needed health care. Risk HMOs are emerging as the preferred kind of Medicare HMO for delivering high quality, cost-effective care to Medicare beneficiaries. Risk plans require that the member obtain all care through the HMO provider network, except in emergencies or upon referral. They offer the lowest out-of-pocket expenses and the lowest premiums. All deductibles and coinsurance are covered, and there are no claim forms to complete in most cases.

•

To summarize this chapter, while HMO benefits can vary from plan to plan and from state to state, basic HMO coverage is fairly consistent across plans because of federal qualification and market competition. Benefit plans vary most in the levels of copayments charged, rather than the scope of services covered.

HMOs offer employers flexibility through special products, such as multiple option plans (MOPs) and point-of-service (POS) plans, that can provide coverage for employees outside of the HMO service area, and allow employees to become gradually accustomed to managed care.

COBRA and individual conversion plans permit people to continue their HMO coverage, rather than lose coverage because of a layoff or family situation. Retirees with Medicare can be covered through several special plans – supplements that wrap around the member's Medicare coverage, or low-cost Medicare risk plans through which the HMO administers the member's Medicare benefits.

7. The Cost of Coverage

Health coverage involves two kind of costs – the *premium* – the cost of the coverage itself – and the *out-of-pocket expenses* involved in obtaining covered care. This chapter examines these two characteristics of health coverage, and how they affect members of HMOs.

Premiums and Out-of-Pocket Costs

For many years, the total cost of the premium was paid by the employer. Recently, it has become more common for employers to pay only a part of the premium and require their employees to make up the difference. For example, an employer may decide to contribute an amount equal to 75% of the employee's premium. The remaining portion, paid by the employee, is called the *employee contribution.*

Out-of-pocket costs are a factor because health plans do not provide *first-dollar coverage*; i.e., 100% coverage of all charges for all services. Instead, a variety of financial incentives, such as copayments, deductibles and coinsurance, may be used to encourage enrollees to seek care only when they really need it. These are the most common kinds of out-of-pocket costs, and they must be considered together with the premium to determine the real value of health insurance coverage.

Deductibles

The *deductible* is a common feature of traditional health insurance coverage. It is a specific level of medical expense that must be paid by an insured person before any payments from the insurance company begin. The amount of the deductible is specified in the person's coverage contract and renews each year. At the point that the insured has paid out the specified amount, it is said that the deductible has been *met* or *satisfied.*

The deductible may also be cumulative among family members so that the deductible is satisfied sooner. For example, an insurance plan may require annual deductibles of $200 per person or $500 per family. Each individual's deductible is met when he or she has paid $200 in expenses, while the deductibles for all family members are met when the family's combined expenses equal $500.

In theory, the deductible gives enrollees a financial incentive to limit the use of services to those that are strictly necessary. In practice, the deductible may actually encourage the patient to obtain services in order to satisfy the deductible requirement so that benefit payments can begin. Deductibles are used mainly by indemnity insurers and PPOs. They are not used by HMOs, but may be found in the indemnity options of hybrid products such as POS plans. Common deductible levels are $250, $500 and $1,000 per year; plans with higher deductibles cost less.

Coinsurance

Coinsurance is a term used to describe the enrollee's share of cost. With this form of coverage, the insurer pays a fixed percentage of the enrollee's medical expenses, and the enrollee pays the balance. It is strongly linked to fee-for-service reimbursement and, as we shall see, shifts some of the insurance risk back onto the insured person.

Coinsurance is usually expressed as a percentage of the *maximum allowed charge (MAC)* or *usual, customary and reasonable (UCR) charge* for a given medical procedure.

Mr. Smith has an earache and indemnity insurance that pays "80% of allowed charges." His family doctor sees him for a brief visit. In the health care industry, this brief visit is represented by the procedure code "99211", for which the doctor's normal charge is $44.00. The physician's office then sends a claim to the patient's insurance company for a 99211 service with a billed charge of $44.00.

The insurance company's maximum allowed charge for the 99211 procedure is $35.00. The insurer compares the doctor's charge of $44.00 with its maximum allowed charge of $35.00, then uses the lower of the two figures to determine the payable amount:

$35.00 X 80% = $28.00

The claim is adjudicated at 80% of the maximum allowable charge. The insurance company will pay $28.00 and Mr. Smith will have to pay the balance of $16.00.

Figure 4. Coinsurance

In a coinsurance system, the insurer establishes a MAC that it will pay for any given procedure. These maximums are developed from surveys of the average charges in the community for each procedure. The maximum is then used by the insurer as the basis for calculating the payable amount and the coinsurance portion. Figure 4 illustrates the effects of coinsurance.

In most cases, the insurer's MAC is less than the provider's billed charge. In the example in Figure 4, the actual rate of coverage is less than the 80% implied by the policy. The insurer actually pays about 64% of the bill in this case, while the patient must pay coinsurance of $16.00 (36% of the total.) In this way, some of the financial risk for care is transferred back onto the patient.

When coinsurance is used in HMOs, the member is responsible for a specific percentage of the HMO's cost, rather than for the remainder of the provider's charge. He or she gets the benefit of the HMO's contracted rates, and the member's out-of-pocket costs for the service are lower than would be the case with indemnity coverage.

With coinsurance, the patient has a financial incentive to use services only when needed because the patient's share increases directly in proportion to the charges for those services. However, coinsurance is a rather poor utilization control strategy because the patient seldom knows the cost of services until after they have been provided. Coinsurance is most common in indemnity plans and PPOs; HMOs use the method only rarely, and then only for certain benefits.

Coinsurance is easy to administer for insurers and is well-understood by health care providers. It has two principal disadvantages: first, out-of-pocket costs are unpredictable because they increase with the number and price of the services performed; second, the fee-for-service basis for reimbursement creates an incentive for providers to perform more services and services of greater complexity in order to increase their revenues. This, in turn, increases the cost to both the patient and the insurer.

Copayments

Copayments are fixed dollar amounts that an enrollee pays directly to a provider at the time of receiving care. Copayments are often used in HMOs for services in which the enrollee can initiate utilization (although not always). Copayments differ according to the kind of service, and the enrollee pays the same copayment amount each time a given service is received.

Typically, only one copayment is charged per visit, even though several different services may be provided. The following are examples of services for which many HMO plan designs require copayments, along with common copayment amounts:

Physician office visits...$5, 10 or 15

Emergency room visits...$25 or 50

Annual physical exams...$15 or 25

Hospital admissions...............................$0, 100, 250 or 500

Prescription drugs...$5, 7 or 9

Mental health visits...$25 or 40

The level of copayments is a feature of the benefit plan chosen by the employer. Premiums for benefit plans with higher copayments are less than premiums for plans with low copayments.

Like deductibles and coinsurance, copayments are intended to reduce unnecessary utilization. However, they can also be structured to encourage utilization. For instance, preventive services such as well baby checkups are often covered with no or low copayments to encourage members to obtain them.

Copayment-based systems also limit out-of-pocket expenses for the enrollee. Unlike coinsurance, the copayment doesn't increase in proportion to the provider's charges, and varies less with the complexity of the services provided. In federally-qualified HMOs, a federal regulation restricts the total annual amount of copayments for which an enrollee may be liable (see page 63.)

How HMOs Set Premium Rates

The rates that employers and individuals pay for HMO coverage are set through a process called *rate setting* or *underwriting*. In this process, the HMO tries to estimate the cost of providing a particular set of benefits so that premiums will be adequate to cover expenses. This section examines some of the issues involved.

Moral Hazard and Adverse Selection

Moral hazard is a term used to describe a situation in which people obtain insurance coverage only at the point when they know they're going to need it. *Adverse selection* is a circumstance in which people select a particular coverage or insurer for some immediate advantage and expose the insurer to unusually high risk in doing so. When a person enrolls for health coverage under either of these conditions, the premiums paid for coverage are rarely sufficient to cover the insurer's costs of treating the condition which prompted the person to enroll.

To protect themselves against moral hazard and adverse selection, insurers try to identify *pre-existing conditions;* i.e., medical conditions or illnesses which an individual has prior to enrolling and which are often the main reason for seeking coverage in the first place. Many indemnity insurers and some HMOs limit or exclude coverage of pre-existing conditions.

As an alternative to pre-existing condition exclusions, some insurers use a *waiting period* to limit benefits during the initial period of coverage, usually ranging from 60 to 180 days. While this strategy limits the insurer's financial exposure, it also prevents the member from receiving comprehensive care until after the waiting period.

Health questionnaires and *medical examinations* are the most common methods of obtaining information for evaluating the risk involved in providing health coverage to an applicant. In HMOs, these methods are limited to calculating initial rates for small group and individual coverage.

Depending on the individual insurer's policies, information from questionnaires or medical exams may be used for a number of purposes – to determine if an individual should be refused coverage, to exclude a particular medical condition from coverage, or to adjust premium rates to compensate for higher-than-average risk.

Federally-qualified HMOs are not permitted to use pre-existing condition exclusions or waiting periods, except in coverage for individuals and for employer groups with less than three employees. HMOs are permitted, however, to use information from health questionnaires and examinations to make adjustments in premiums for new groups based on their risk factors (see next section.) This medical information is considered along with census data in the rate setting process in some HMOs.

Rating and Underwriting

Many federally-qualified HMOs use a process called *community rating* to set premium rates for employer groups. With community rating, premiums are based on the average cost of providing care to the HMO's enrollees. An alternate rating method, *adjusted community rating,* starts with the community rate and then permits the rate for a prospective or renewing group to be adjusted for anticipated utilization. To make this adjustment, HMO underwriters evaluate the demographic characteristics of the group and try to forecast the group's utilization of medical services based on various risk factors. *Risk factors* are characteristics that are statistically correlated with higher than average use of health services, such as the age and sex composition of the group's employees, type of business, and number of years in operation.

Experience rating is the rating method used by most traditional indemnity insurers, and by some non-federally-qualified HMOs. With experience rating, rates are based mostly on the employer group's utilization characteristics or claims experience, without regard to the utilization or expense characteristics of the insurer's groups as a whole.

Compared with traditional insurance, HMO rate setting practices tend to promote access to health care. Since most HMOs use some variation of community rating, their premiums are more consistent from group to group than insurance premiums based on experience rating. Also, federally-qualified HMOs are not permitted to use pre-existing condition exclusions or waiting periods for groups of three or more individuals, and must offer annual open enrollment periods. As a result, HMOs offer improved access to care for those who otherwise might be unable to obtain health coverage.

Premium Structure

Once the basic premiums have been set for a specific employer group, premiums are determined for each *family size* or *tier type*. The following are some examples:

3-Tier Rating

employee only ('single') $110
employee plus spouse ('double') $220
employee, spouse and children ('family')...................$385

4-Tier Rating

employee only ('single') $110
employee plus spouse ('double') $220
employee plus children ('single plus children') $275
employee, spouse and children ('family')...................$385

In this approach, the premium to be charged for each employee is based on the employee's family size. When a subscriber or family member has Medicare as the primary coverage, many HMOs give a discount called a *Medicare offset* as a deduction from the member's premium. This discount is given because the HMO's potential liability is somewhat reduced by the member's Medicare coverage. Offsets are not normally offered for members covered by another insurance plan other than Medicare.

Do You Have Dual Coverage?

These days, it is not unusual for people to be covered by more than one health insurance, especially in families where the subscriber and spouse both work. This situation, called *dual coverage,* creates two issues of which consumers should be aware. First, in a process called *coordination of benefits (COB),* HMOs coordinate their benefit payments with the member's other insurance coverage so that the provider is not paid more than the total of the member's medical bill.

Insurance companies and HMOs use a set of COB rules to determine which plan is the *primary insurer* and which is *secondary insurer.* The primary insurer pays first, and any remaining amounts are paid by the secondary plan. This process usually takes place without having to involve the member directly.

However, as a consumer, the member does have a direct interest in the potential cost of maintaining dual coverage. Indemnity plans have a high out-of-pocket cost, so dual coverage may make sense for people with an indemnity policy. On the other hand, HMO coverage is comprehensive enough that it leaves little out-of-pocket expense for a second insurance plan to cover, so dual coverage is often a waste of money.

For people with dual coverage, there are three factors to consider. In most cases, they would want to drop the health plan with the lesser benefits if: 1) doing so would save them money or increase the funds available for other options in an employee flexible benefits plan; 2) the family could keep the plan with the better benefits; and 3) there are no obstacles to regaining the lost coverage should circumstances change (job layoff, divorce, etc.) If you have dual coverage, you may wish to explore the options with your benefits manager or personnel department.

8. How HMOs Pay Providers

Methods of Payment

HMO enrollees may receive health care services from a wide variety of providers who contract with or work for the HMO. The number of contracting provider relationships is especially great in IPA and network model HMOs, and the method used to pay a given claim is determined by the contractual relationship. When care is received from a contracting provider, payment may be made in several ways.

Retrospective Payment

Retrospective payment methods, such as fee schedules and discounted fee-for-service, reimburse providers for services after the services have been rendered. Under such arrangements, when enrollees obtain services for which the HMO is financially responsible, the provider sends a claim form to the HMO. The HMO then reviews the claim to ensure that several conditions have been met:

- The patient was enrolled on the date of service

- Any required authorization was obtained

- The service was medically necessary

- The service is covered by the enrollee's benefit plan

If the claim passes this review, the provider is paid at the payment rates specified in the contract. If more information is required, the claim may be *suspended* (placed on hold) until additional records are received from the provider to substantiate the need for the services.

Most providers prefer payment by retrospective methods because these methods are familiar, owing to their wide use by indemnity insurance carriers. However, the retrospective approach pays providers a separate fee for each service performed, giving providers an incentive to furnish more care than may be necessary. By performing more procedures or procedures of greater complexity, providers can increase the payment they receive. When used in HMOs, retrospective payment is paired with utilization management systems to counter this incentive to over-utilize services. Whenever possible, HMOs try to avoid the incentives of retrospective payment by using contracts based on prospective payment.

Prospective Payment

HMOs emphasize prospective payment methods because prospective payment does the most to encourage preventive care and control costs. The most common method of prospective payment is called *capitation.* HMOs tend to use capitation to pay providers for high-volume services for which the provider is willing to accept a degree of financial risk, such as physician, laboratory, or hospital care.

In a capitation arrangement, a provider is paid in advance (prospectively) to provide a specific range of medical services to a specific subset of HMO enrollees. Capitation is analogous to the premium paid by an employer group to the HMO in that it is a prepayment; in this case, though, the HMO pays capitation to a provider to furnish a specific subset of health services.

The HMO pays the capitated provider a fixed amount each month for each of the provider's assigned HMO enrollees *(per member per month* or *pmpm),* regardless of how much or how little it actually costs the provider to care for those enrollees. The capitation payment can be thought of as a budget out of which all expenses incurred by the provider must be paid. If expenses are less than the capitation payments, then the provider makes money; if expenses exceed capitation, the provider loses money. This is the risk that HMOs and providers take on in providing health care on a prepaid basis.

The risks of capitation create two incentives for providers: first, to render only services that are necessary, as the provider must absorb or pay the cost of those services; and second, to furnish preventive services that keep enrollees healthy, because preventive services that maintain health cost less than therapeutic services for treating illness.

Under a capitation agreement, the question of who pays a claim can become rather complex. Each service provided to a member is the responsibility of either the HMO or the capitated provider. Typically, a physician group is capitated for services that its member physicians can control. These include professional services from physicians, surgeons and therapists, and outpatient services such as radiology, laboratory, ambulatory surgery, etc. The HMO retains responsibility for services over which physicians have less direct influence, such as hospital and emergency room facility charges, and ancillary services such as ambulance, home health and durable medical equipment.

The contract with the provider must specify those services that are the financial responsibility of the provider under the capitation arrangement. Services that are not listed are presumed to be the responsibility of the HMO. The manner in which this separation of financial responsibility is maintained is discussed further in the next section.

Paying for Physician Services

In managed-care jargon, a visit to the doctor is called an *encounter*. Encounters are categorized as brief, intermediate, comprehensive, etc., depending on the length of time spent with the patient and the scope of the examination. To see how these services are paid, let's first look at the case of physician encounters in a staff or group model HMO.

Encounters – Staff/Group Model

When an encounter takes place in an HMO or medical group facility, no bill or claim form is generated. Instead, an *encounter form* is used to record the services received by the patient. Encounter information is entered into a computer system for tracking patient data and physician productivity. While the encounter does have a real cost, that cost is borne internally by the HMO or medical group; the physician typically receives no payment for the encounter itself because he or she is on salary (another form of prospective payment) or shares in the group's profits through a partnership interest.

Encounters – IPA/Network Model

Encounters in an IPA or network setting can be paid prospectively or retrospectively. In a prospective arrangement, the HMO pays for physician care with a capitation payment to the medical group. When paying retrospectively, it uses a variation of the fee-for-service method. But how are individual doctors in an IPA or medical group paid for the care they provide?

Figure 5 illustrates the payment relationships between the HMO, the IPA and the IPA physicians. In the diagram, the

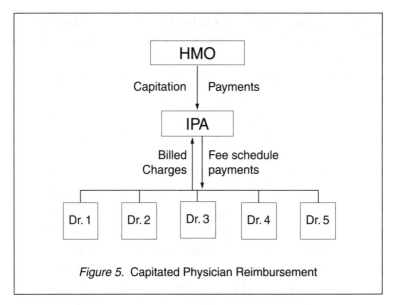

Figure 5. Capitated Physician Reimbursement

HMO makes a monthly capitation payment to the physicians group, a fixed amount per member per month of coverage. The payment is made at the beginning of each month as prepayment of all services to be rendered by the IPA physicians in the month ahead.

The IPA, in turn, may pay its member physicians in a number of ways. The most common methods parallel the retrospective method used by physicians in their general practice, i.e., fee-for-service reimbursement. As physicians provide services to HMO enrollees, they send bills with their standard charges to the IPA. In a *discounted fee-for-service* arrangement, the IPA then deducts a standard percentage from the charge for each service and pays the doctor the reduced amount. Alternatively, the physician group may pay each procedure using a *fee schedule,* a table of customary rates paid to members of the group. With this method, a given procedure is always paid at the same rate, regardless of the physician's original charge.

Some medical groups provide their PCPs with additional compensation to encourage them to actively manage care for their enrollees. This approach pays the PCP something extra for the effort involved in following up on specialist referrals, lab tests and treatments. In some arrangements, case management incentive payments take the form of extra payments made for each claim a PCP submits.

In some IPA and network HMOs, physician groups capitate their PCPs to encourage case management. In PCP capitation, the PCP receives a fixed amount per member per month for each member in his or her panel. PCP capitation funds come from the larger capitation payment made by the HMO to the physicians group. PCP capitation arrangements are controversial because they give the PCP an incentive to try to provide all of a member's care in order to minimize referrals. Many experts feel that it is best to have capitation at the medical group/IPA level, paired with fee schedule reimbursement of individual physicians.

Split Responsibility Claims

Provider contracts must try to anticipate the complexity of real life situations. For example, patients treated in the hospital often receive many different kinds of services. In its capitation contract with the HMO, the medical group is responsible for certain services while the HMO is liable for others. Staff and group-model HMOs can deal with this shared financial responsibility with straightforward accounting, as the HMO and physician administrative functions are well integrated and most care is provided in-house. However, in IPA and network HMOs, HMO and medical group are more separated, and coordination of this split financial responsibility is not as easy. To see why, let's review the scenario shown in Figure 6.

```
           Community Hospital
         Statement of Patient Account

Department                          Charge

Cardiology                            $253
Emergency room                        $474
Hospital ward                       $1,400
Laboratory                            $620
Radiology                             $547
Central Supply                         $98

Total charges                       $3,392
```

Figure 6. Split Responsibility Claim

This hospital bill lists charges for services rendered to an
HMO member. In this example, the medical group/HMO
contract provides that charges for inpatient hospital services are the responsibility of the HMO, while charges for
emergency room services are payable by the medical
group. The hospital sends the bill to the HMO, where
claims staff review the bill to determine eligibility and
medical necessity, and identify services for which the
HMO is responsible. These are approved for payment; the
emergency room charge, however, is denied.

A check and a document called a *remittance advice* are
sent to the hospital to pay the claim. The remittance advice
tells the hospital which services are being paid and at what
rate, based on the HMO's contract with the hospital. The
denied emergency charge – for which the medical group is
responsible – has a notation that informs the hospital that
the bill has been sent to the medical group for payment.

At the medical group, the bill is reviewed and the emergency room charge paid. In some cases, the medical group may have a contract with the hospital, and pays its portion at contracted rates. In a sense, the medical group functions as a second insurer, covering the services for which it has been capitated by the HMO.

The issue of shared financial responsibility is presented here because HMO members should know that their treatment may be paid for by several entities. This shared responsibility can occur in many situations where complex care is provided, such as emergency room, outpatient surgery and hospital care. The contracting provider – in this case, the hospital – agrees to accept the HMO and medical group payments, together with any applicable member copayment, as payment in full; the member is not required to pay any balance due.

Paying for Hospital Services

While some staff and group-model HMOs operate their own hospitals, most HMOs contract with hospitals in the community to provide acute care services. Like physician groups, these contracting hospitals give discounts to HMOs in anticipation of increasing or maintaining patient volume. There are five common methods of paying for hospital services.

❏ The most common method of payment for inpatient hospital services in IPA and network HMOs is the *per diem* rate, Latin for "per day". Per diems are negotiated in advance and are related to the average charge for a day in the hospital. They cover all services provided to the patient, no matter how many services are used or what those services may actually cost in an individual case. The patient incurs a per diem charge for each day spent in the hospital, and the bill increases in proportion to the length of the hospital stay.

❏ Using the *discounted charges* method, the HMO receives a straight percentage discount off each bill, usually in the range of ten to twenty percent. HMO provider contracts with hospitals often use different methods to pay for inpatient and outpatient services. While the discounted charges method is sometimes used to pay for inpatient services, it is most widely used for outpatient services. This retrospective method is identical to discounted charges arrangements made with physicians and ancillary providers.

❏ *Case rates* or *global rates* are often negotiated for specific procedures or diagnoses, such as cardiac bypass surgery or maternity care. With this payment method, the patient receives all necessary care for a fixed charge, regardless of the length of stay in the hospital or the amount or cost of resources used. Case rates may be negotiated in advance as part of a provider contract, or on an individual basis as needed.

❏ Hospitals can be paid through *capitation arrangements* to provide all necessary hospital services to a specific group of HMO members. This payment method is common in group model HMOs, and in network plans for members who select PCPs in a particular medical group or IPA affiliated with the hospital. Capitation is calculated by the same methods used for physician capitation.

In one type of capitation arrangement, a hospital and its physicians join together in a *physician-hospital organization (PHO)*. The PHO functions as a contracting representative in negotiations with HMOs and other managed-care organizations. The PHO allows the hospital and its medical staff to assume virtually all of the risk for providing care to a group of patients and helps preserve the hospital's market share by "locking in" the capitated membership.

❑ *Diagnostic-related groups (DRGs)* are used by some HMOs to pay for hospital care. This system, designed for use in the Medicare program, categorizes patients into groups based on diagnosis. DRGs assume that the patients in a given diagnostic group require medical services of similar complexity and intensity, and therefore use medical resources at about the same rate.

Although similar to case rates, there is a distinct reimbursement rate and standard length of stay for each of the 468 diagnostic groups. As with case rates, the hospital is paid the same amount regardless of how many services are actually needed to care for the patient. However, the hospital can be paid more if the patient needs to be hospitalized for substantially longer than the length of stay assigned to the DRG.

Paying for Other Services

Most of the methods discussed in this chapter can also be used to pay for "ancillary" services from other kinds of providers, such as ambulance, home care and laboratory. Of those methods, discounted fee-for-service, fee schedules and case rates are the most common. Capitation may be used for some ancillary providers, especially in high-volume services such as laboratory. Payment for a given ancillary service may be the financial responsibility of either the HMO or the medical group.

•

In this chapter, we have discussed the rationale for paying providers on a prospective basis, and some of the methods used by HMOs to reimburse their contracting providers. HMOs try to structure their provider payment arrangements so that providers have financial incentives to emphasize prevention, case management and coordination, and cost-effective care.

9. Quality of Care in HMOs

As with other innovations, there are skeptics who remain suspicious of HMOs and managed care. Implicit in many of the comments from this quarter seems to be one basic question: is the quality of health care provided by HMOs equal to that provided through the traditional health care system? Before we attempt to answer this question, it will be worthwhile to explore some of the subtleties of this debate.

First, the term "quality" must be defined. Within the health-care community, there is intense interest in the definition and measurement of quality, and the specific standards of quality to which HMOs should be held. A person with a clinical orientation will tend to see quality in terms of health indicators such as immunization rates or the number of women receiving prenatal care.

On the other hand, a consumer advocate may evaluate quality using measures such as the average waiting time for an appointment, and overall member satisfaction. Depending on a given individual's point of view, different definitions of quality will result. These different definitions all have some validity; in response, many HMOs now document their performance in a range of quality areas.

Underlying much of the discussion about the quality of care in HMOs are some assumptions about the methods they use to reimburse health care providers. First, there is an assumption that, because provider incentives are different when treating HMO members, the quality of care must somehow suffer when compared to the quality of care provided through the fee-for-service environment.

There is a limited basis for this argument. Prospective payment methods such as capitation do change provider incentives and modify the practice behavior found in the fee-for-service environment. As a result, prepaid HMO settings may give some providers an incentive to provide less care.

Therefore, HMOs must monitor their providers to ensure that referral and preventive care services are being provided according to regulatory and HMO standards. However, as noted previously, this incentive to limit care is also countered by the larger incentive for providers to give people the care they need to keep them well.

The argument against prepayment also fails to account for the fact that traditional quality management mechanisms in the health care industry are operational for HMO members, too, and that the processes for promoting quality care in HMOs actually complement those traditional processes already established present in the health care system.

For example, a board-certified physician is just as certified for HMO patients as for fee-for-service patients; a hospital accredited by the Joint Commission on the Accreditation of Healthcare Organizations (JCAHO) is accredited for all patients, regardless of who pays the bill.

The quality question then must be considered in the context of these processes already functioning in the health care system at the provider level. HMO members benefit from these external quality mechanisms – board certification of physicians, hospital accreditation programs, credentialing of physicians for hospital privileges, and Medicare certification – as much as patients seen through any other insurance arrangement.

On the other hand, it is HMO members who have a quality advantage. HMOs are required to maintain an additional layer of quality review under federal regulations and the laws of most states. These additional safeguards are not present for people covered by traditional insurance because indemnity insurers are not legally required to monitor the quality of care rendered by providers. Therefore, HMO members benefit from quality systems at two levels – those traditional processes in the health care system and those within the HMO itself.

The utilization review (UR) systems found in HMOs also reinforce quality health care because their authorization and concurrent review processes makes it difficult for doctors to treat patients in isolation. Major therapeutic decisions are routinely reviewed by a third party – an HMO medical director or UR nurse – who is familiar with prevailing standards of medical practice. As a result of this review, there is less chance that the patient will receive inappropriate treatment due to physician error or inexperience.

Returning to the question of whether or not HMOs provide quality care, a number of recent independent studies (see references on page 115) have examined indicators of quality such as clinical outcomes, utilization of preventive services and member satisfaction. They conclude that HMOs provide care which is at least as good as, if not better than, care available through the traditional fee-for-service medical care system.

HMO quality management (QM) programs are implemented in a variety of ways. In the pages that follow, we will examine some of the common systems used by HMOs to monitor and improve the quality of their health care. Virtually all HMOs have most of these systems in place.

Medical Quality Management

Formal *quality management* or *quality improvement* programs in HMOs are designed to provide ongoing evaluation of the quality of health care received by HMO members. Large HMOs have special departments devoted to this function, while smaller HMOs may use staff from the Utilization Review or Medical Affairs departments to conduct QM activities. The HMO's medical director or medical vice president has overall responsibility for the quality management program.

Due to the large number of contracted providers involved in many HMOs, QM programs must deal with considerable organizational and political complexity. Most contracting hospitals and physician groups have their own quality management system, quality committees and QM staff. The HMO's QM system must work together with these other systems to promote the particular quality goals of the HMO.

Most HMOs find that a committee structure works best for involving the various parties interested in the QM process. Through a committee, it is possible to create a consensus for decisions and recommendations, and obtain cooperation for their implementation. In staff and group-model HMOs, the QM committee often consists of representatives from various clinical specialties such as family practice, nursing, laboratory, surgery, and home care. In IPA and network-model plans, representatives from the HMO's physicians group are included to ensure that QM activities are uniformly implemented for all plan members.

Depending on the HMO, a number of functions may fall within the scope of the quality management program, including retrospective review, technology assessment, and the standards of care program. The QM committee also may play a significant role in the appeals process (see Grievance and Appeals Systems on page 107.)

Quality Management Studies

Quality management studies or audits are the most common means of evaluating the quality of care in HMOs. On an ongoing basis, the QM committee devises retrospective studies of some aspect of clinical practice in the HMO. Commonly, these studies evaluate the plan's compliance with standards or recommendations for screening exams and preventive procedures issued by recognized authorities, such as the American Academy of Pediatrics or the National Institutes of Health.

Data for QM studies may be obtained from encounters, claims, utilization review notes or medical records. Common areas of study include childhood immunization rates, the percentage of women over age fifty receiving mammograms in the past year, the percentage of members receiving a physical exam in the last year, and the percentage of patients discharged from a hospital and re-admitted within thirty days.

Here's an example of how such a review might be structured. An HMO decides to evaluate its performance in immunizing children in comparison to national averages. Its QM staff conduct a review of the medical records of a sample of the plan's pediatricians. The rates of immunization for children in the HMO are determined and then compared with the national average.

When the data are analyzed and summarized, findings are reviewed by members of the QM committee, and then published and distributed to plan physicians. Based on the findings, the committee may take a number of steps, including making recommendations for changes in HMO medical policies, designating certain problem providers for intensive review or monitoring, and creating educational programs to increase providers' overall compliance with standards.

Technology Assessment

Many HMOs have a *technology assessment* department which evaluates the relative effectiveness of surgical procedures, medical treatments, drugs and devices. Information obtained through this process enhances the overall quality of care provided by the HMO in several ways.

Technology assessment is conducted primarily through literature reviews; surveys of specialists and experts; and searches of medical and pharmaceutical on-line databases. Using these tools, physicians, nurses and/or medical librarians collect and assimilate the latest information available on a given subject. Researchers may incorporate findings from sources such as journals, Medicare coverage manuals and reports from government agencies such as the Food & Drug Administration and Centers for Disease Control.

On an immediate basis, technology assessment information may be used in authorization review to help determine whether a request should be approved. Over the long term, results of research influence the plan's medical policy and help determine whether certain treatments become covered benefits. Technology assessment also plays an important role in determining standards of care (see below) and in the design and performance of quality management studies.

Standards of Care

Some HMOs develop formal policies for the treatment of specific diseases and conditions, and for preventive and primary care. These *standards of care*, or *treatment protocols,* can be developed for those clinical areas of medical practice where the diagnostic and therapeutic approaches are well-defined and generally accepted.

Using information derived from technology assessment research, quality studies and participating specialists, standards are established for a particular disease. The standards set forth the kind and sequence of diagnostic tests and procedures needed to confirm a certain diagnosis, and the established procedures and drug therapies to be used in treating the condition.

Once standards are in place, physicians in the HMO's contracting medical groups are educated as to the use of the standards and may be expected to follow them. Standards of care have great potential for bringing physician practice up to the "state of the art". By standardizing physicians on the most effective proven treatments, the HMO can have a significant educational influence on its physicians and improve the quality of care for all its members.

Provider Credentialing

Provider credentialing is a process through which the HMO reviews a provider's qualifications prior to becoming part of the HMO network. Outside of HMOs, readers may be familiar with the credentialing process used by hospitals when a physician applies for admitting privileges. In this process, the physician's credentials are reviewed and verified by the hospital: possession of a valid medical license, graduation from medical school, completion of an approved residency and specialty board examination, if applicable; and a search of practitioner databanks to discover any history of malpractice problems or sanctions.

It is interesting that many credentialing processes rely on a series of indirect or proxy indicators to assess a provider's competence, instead of on direct measures. Most health care organizations, including HMOs, use similar proxy measures to determine the qualifications because direct measures have not been readily available. That situation appears to be changing though, due to a growing emphasis on measuring the outcomes of patient care in institutions and HMOs (see HMO Report Cards and Accreditation on page 111.)

In many HMOs, credentialing of IPAs and medical groups is similar to a hospital credentialing process, in terms of the kinds of information reviewed for each physician in the group. Credentialing of other providers, such as laboratories, hospitals and home care agencies, is done by obtaining equivalent information, such as state license number, Medicare certification, and JCAHO accreditation status. Also, the financial status of a provider may be reviewed to determine that the provider can sustain a long-term relationship with the HMO, particularly when capitation or other risk-sharing is involved.

In addition to verifying the provider's qualifications, many HMOs supplement their credentialing reviews with facility site reviews. The HMO may evaluate characteristics of the provider's facility, such as accessibility, appearance, organization and cleanliness. HMO staff may check to see if office hours are posted, or analyze the waiting times for various kinds of appointments. The plan may review the qualifications of the provider's clinical staff, and check the provider's compliance with guidelines for instrument sterilization, medication storage and infectious waste disposal.

An HMO credentials its providers not only to ensure high quality care, but also because credentialing helps sell the plan in the marketplace. The HMO's provider network is one of its most important assets; a large percentage of board-certified physicians and Medicare-certified ancillary providers are important factors in attracting membership. Accessible, well-run provider facilities mean that members are more likely to be satisfied with their care and have less reason to switch to another HMO. Through credentialing programs, HMOs can assure prospective members of the quality of their providers in a way that traditional insurance carriers cannot.

Grievance and Appeals Systems

HMOs have formal grievance and appeals systems to resolve member complaints. These dispute resolution systems are required for federally-qualified HMOs and by many states. *Grievance systems* may be used to hear complaints about an HMO's administrative procedures and performance issues, while *appeal processes* are used when an HMO denies a member's request for coverage of a medical service. While they provide the enrollee with a forum in which to question the HMO's policies and decisions, these systems are also an important source of feedback to plan administrators and quality management programs.

The Grievance System

In a typical HMO grievance system, member complaints are reviewed by a series of committees. The process starts when a member contacts the HMO's Member Services department to lodge a complaint. If the complaint cannot be resolved to the member's satisfaction by Member Services staff, the member may file a formal grievance by writing a letter to the HMO or by completing a special grievance form. In the grievance document, the member describes the nature of the problem, the attempts taken so far to resolve the problem, and the member's view on how the problem should be resolved.

Upon receipt by the HMO, the grievance is heard at the next meeting of the plan's *Grievance Committee*. This committee meets every month or as needed, and is composed of representatives from the HMO's major departments. The committee reviews the member's written grievance as it relates to the HMO's policies and the member's terms of coverage. Based on this review, the committee can rule in favor of the member or sustain the original finding. The decision is then communicated to the member along with the HMO's proposed resolution.

If the member isn't satisfied with the committee's decision, he or she may make a written request for a rehearing of the decision. A second committee is convened, composed of members of the health plan's senior management staff or its Board of Directors. The facts of the case are reviewed, and the committee either reaches a decision in favor of the member or upholds the original decision. The member is then notified of the results of the re-hearing.

In some plans, the second-level committee makes the final decision. However, most grievance systems allow for additional levels of appeal, including binding arbitration or civil court proceedings at the highest level.

The Appeal Process

While grievances deal with administrative and procedural issues, appeals are concerned with coverage and benefit decisions. When the HMO or contracting medical group denies a request for a medical service, the member may appeal that denial through the appeals process. The member writes a letter stating why he or she believes the service should be covered, and may include medical records or documentation from a physician.

As with grievances, the appeal is typically reviewed by a committee of doctors and nurses. The committee examines the request for consistency with the HMO's criteria, and the member's benefits and terms of coverage. Based on this review, the committee may find in favor of the member or uphold the original denial. The member is notified of the committee's decision and given an opportunity to respond.

Additional hearings may be possible, and some systems permit the member to present his or her case in person or to be accompanied by legal representation at the appeal level. Members of Medicare plans have several additional levels of appeal through HCFA and the courts. While the details of HMO grievance and appeal systems vary widely from plan to plan and from state to state, all are designed to make the HMO responsive to its consumers, and to give the member a means of challenging the HMO bureaucracy.

Assessing Member Satisfaction

Many HMOs conduct *member satisfaction surveys* to determine if members are satisfied with the HMO's services. These surveys are taken annually and serve several purposes: they may identify problem areas where the plan needs to improve its operations, they can call attention to access or quality problems with particular providers, and they generally give the plan feedback on how it is perceived by its enrollees.

Member surveys are usually administered in one of two forms, either as written questionnaires or by telephone. The survey is administered to a portion of the HMO's membership. The responses of this representative sample are analyzed to understand the opinions of the general membership.

Membership satisfaction surveys can cover a wide variety of topics. Each survey question is designed so that the respondent evaluates some aspect of the HMO's performance. These are some frequently asked questions:

- Have you had a physical exam since joining the plan?

- Have you changed PCPs in the last year? Why?

- Have you ever been a member of any other HMO?

- How easy or difficult did you find it to select a PCP?

- What factors influenced you to join the HMO?

- How long did you have to wait for your last appointment?

- Have you ever had to contact your physician after-hours?

- Have you ever felt it necessary to use a non-plan provider?

- Have you ever received the plan's newsletter?

- Do you feel that the HMO's telephone system is adequate?

- Does the health plan provide you with enough information on how to use its services?

- Would you recommend the HMO to your friends?

Satisfaction surveys measure what could be called the administrative and subjective components of quality as experienced by the individual enrollee. These include such factors as patient convenience, accessibility of providers, and courtesy of office staff and health plan representatives.

Summarized data are used mainly in two ways. Areas in which the plan scores poorly can become the subject for further review by the HMO and its quality review program. Those areas in which the HMO scores well may be used to differentiate the plan from its competition and to promote it in marketing presentations and advertising.

HMO Report Cards

The idea of publishing *HMO report cards,* which disclose an HMO's performance relative to various standards, has recently gained considerable popularity. Although not yet widely available, employers will eventually use them to compare the relative performance and effectiveness of competing HMOs. Summary versions will be available to individuals to assist them in choosing an HMO.

While several large HMOs have begun to produce report cards, the most ambitious attempt at standardized reporting to date is the *Health Plan Employer Data and Information Set (HEDIS)*. HEDIS was designed by a coalition of representatives from major HMOs and leading national employers. It is the most comprehensive reporting model yet developed for evaluating the performance of managed-care organizations.

HEDIS is essentially a reporting system which defines a set of *quality measures* (performance indicators) for the HMO industry, and standardizes the methods used to report those measures. Each HMO would produce its own report card on a periodic basis, organizing its information according to the HEDIS standards, and comparing its performance with national norms in each of the standard quality areas.

HEDIS brings together clinical indicators and member satisfaction data along with other indicators such as utilization statistics and financial performance. The following is a summary of the quality measures used by HEDIS:

- **Clinical indicators** include performance in preventive services, prenatal care, acute and chronic illness, mental health and substance abuse

- **Member satisfaction indicators** focus on accessi bility of health services, member satisfaction survey activities and results

- **Utilization indicators** report on utilization rates for inpatient and maternity hospitalization and lengths of stay; ambulatory services, prescription usage and frequency of common surgical procedures; enrollment and disenrollment rates

- **Financial indicators** include premium rate and expense trends, measures of financial stability, protections against financial insolvency

- **Management programs** are described in terms of the HMO's operational and administrative programs

One of the most important aspects of HEDIS is that it specifies the methods that are to be used to report each of the quality measures. Following the HEDIS standards, data are categorized according to the same rules by each HMO and reported in a standard format, thereby facilitating comparison of data from different plans. Furthermore, HEDIS is significant because it represents a shift away from proxy indicators of quality toward indicators based on the outcomes and effectiveness of patient care.

HEDIS data are complex enough so that they may not be immediately useful to an individual trying to decide which HMO to join. Also, HEDIS is an evolving system – its performance indicators will change over time as it expands in scope and refinement. However, even in its present form, HEDIS will increase the ability of large employers to perform meaningful comparisons of HMO performance, and provide a basis for summary report cards oriented toward the HMO consumer and member.

Accreditation of HMOs

Accreditation is a recent development in the trend toward validating the quality of care provided by HMOs. The *National Committee for Quality Assurance (NCQA)* is a non-profit, independent review organization that accredits HMOs. Working with employers, health care providers and HMOs, the NCQA has developed a set of rigorous accreditation standards that it uses in evaluating HMO programs. There is no comparable quality evaluation program for fee-for-service health care.

NCQA accreditation is a voluntary accreditation process that focuses on HMO operations in several key areas – quality management, utilization management, provider credentialing, member rights and responsibilities, preventive care services and medical records. The accreditation process is accomplished through a review of plan documentation and records, on-site surveys and informational staff interviews, and evaluation of member service systems.

Once the review process is complete, the HMO is given an *accreditation status:* full, one-year or provisional accreditation; accreditation denied; or under review. Full accreditation is awarded for three years and does not automatically renew. However, an organization can request a review more often than every three years in order to receive a higher accreditation status.

About one-half of American HMOs have applied for or undergone accreditation through NCQA. The review process is exhaustive and comprehensive, and HMOs will spend a year or more in preparation for the review. NCQA standards complement the regulatory requirements for HMOs; whereas most HMO laws require that HMOs establish and maintain systems in areas such as quality management, member grievance and credentialing, NCQA standards evaluate the actual quality of those processes, their effectiveness and integration into HMO operations.

Though accreditation is relatively new, employers and individual HMO members eventually will come to view it as a basic measure of value and quality. As more HMOs become accredited, it is a certainty that accreditation will become a competitive necessity for HMOs and the standard for the managed-care market.

The drive to validate the quality of care is strong in HMOs, owing in part, perhaps, to a historical need of HMOs to prove themselves. Accreditation, HEDIS and report cards are quality promotion tools that are unique to HMOs – nothing similar is available with traditional indemnity insurers because insurance carriers do not contract with providers and aren't organized into provider networks.

•

The variety of quality management programs reviewed in this chapter demonstrates the decided advantage that HMO members have in the area of quality management and assurance. Quality improvement systems at the provider level are complemented by HMO systems at the network level. No other form of health care organization does more to monitor the quality of care provided to enrollees.

References (from page 101):

Langa KM, Sussman EJ. The Effect of Cost Containment Policies on Rates of Coronary Revascularization in California. *New Engl J Med* 1993; 329(24): 1784-1789.

Carlisle DM, et al. HMO vs. Fee-for-Service Care of Older Persons with Acute Myocardial Infarction. *Am J Pub Hlth* 1992; 82:1626-1630.

Udvarhelyi IS, et al. Comparison of the Quality of Ambulatory Care for Fee-for-Service and Prepaid Patients. *Ann of Int Med* 1991; 115: 394-400.

Brook RH, et al. Quality of Ambulatory Care: Epidemiology and Comparison by Insurance Status and Income. *Medical Care* 1990; 28(5): 392-410.

Valdez RB, et al. Prepaid Group Practice Effects on the Utilization of Medical Services and Health Outcomes for Children: Results of a Randomized Trial. *Pediatrics* 1989; 83(2): 168-180.

Sloss EM, et al. Effect of a Health Maintenance Organization on Physiologic Health: Results from a Randomized Trial. *Ann of Int Med* 1987; 106: 130-138.

---

10. Looking Forward

While our traditional medical care system provides generally excellent care, it does have some significant problems. As we have seen, these problems often result not from the way health care is provided, but from the way that health providers are paid. The system is prone to over-utilization and inefficiency, and lacks coordination. In this *à la carte* system, care may be fragmented among many providers, each of whom has an incentive to maximize reimbursement by providing more services.

HMOs manage care in order to correct the problems we have noted, with the result that care through an HMO costs less without compromises in quality. HMOs are integrated health care systems that use a range of strategies and techniques to improve on undesirable characteristics of traditional health care. Reimbursement strategies work to reduce the provision of unnecessary services; utilization review and case management systems ensure that care is appropriate, effective and coordinated.

Combined with extensive quality improvement programs, these techniques are the building blocks of managed care in HMOs. From the appearance of the first symptoms through convalescence and return to work, care is managed in an organized fashion that promotes quality. This is the real value that HMOs offer to HMO members and employers. With this in mind, this chapter examines two areas with long-term implications for members of HMOs: the role that HMOs may play in national health care reform, and a glimpse of what may lie ahead in the evolution of the HMO model.

National Health Care Reform

The state of the American health care system has become one of the major issues of the 1990s, and may well remain on the domestic policy agenda into the next century.

In spite of its technical excellence, medical care consumes over 14% of the output of the American economy, substantially higher than the 8 to 9% in other developed countries. Access to care, for the most part, is based on having insurance coverage – millions of Americans forego adequate preventive and routine care because they lack health insurance. The system permits some private-sector suppliers to make exorbitant profits, while other providers, such as county hospitals, struggle to survive. The cost to employers of providing insurance has become so high that some employers have stopped contributing to their employees coverage altogether, thereby adding to the problems of access to care.

Many of the managed-care techniques used by HMOs in their day-to-day operations are directed toward the same problems addressed by health care reform proposals at the national level. Furthermore, in taking stock of the health care system, reformers have tried to recognize and build upon those elements of the health care system that work well. It is no surprise that HMOs and managed care are seen as proven solutions to these problems, and have been incorporated into a number of national reform proposals.

While the various reform proposals differ widely in specific details, there are some common themes we can examine. Several of the major proposals are based on the *managed competition* approach. In this approach, health coverage would be provided through *purchasing cooperatives* or *health alliances*. These alliances would be established regionally and function as intermediaries – bringing together many employer groups, on the one hand, with health care providers which we will call *managed-care organizations* or *MCOs*.

On the consumer side, employers would purchase group health coverage through the local cooperative or alliance. Anyone, including individuals, could obtain coverage through the alliance at its standard rates. Benefits would be standardized to a few basic plans, thereby simplifying the process of selecting coverage. Alliances would not be permitted to use experience rating, and alliances and MCOs would have to provide coverage to anyone, even people with pre-existing conditions. As alliance members, employees and individuals could choose to receive care from any of the alliance's contracting health plans.

To provide health care, alliances would contract with a number of selected MCOs. An alliance would use the size of its membership to negotiate the best possible rates with each of its contracting MCOs. Health care services would be provided by the MCOs, and the alliance would administer member eligibility systems, premium collection and other administrative functions.

MCOs would most likely be HMOs and other managed-care organizations, offering their networks of contracting hospitals and physician groups. Figure 7 (on the next page) illustrates the basic structure of a purchasing cooperative or health alliance arrangement.

MCOs would compete for alliance members based on the price of coverage and the quality of their services and providers. To be successful as an alliance provider, an MCO would have to be able to provide high-quality care efficiently and at low cost. Of all the types of health plans

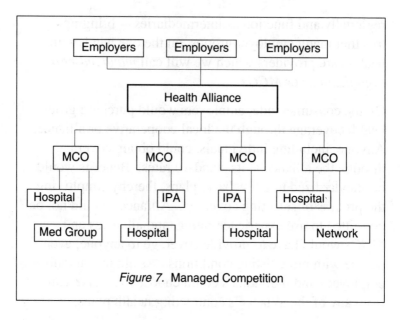

Figure 7. Managed Competition

now in existence, HMOs are the best positioned to begin functioning immediately as MCOs – they are years ahead of the rest of the health care industry in managing care, provider contracting, prospective payment, utilization monitoring and performance reporting.

There is another major health reform model in which the role of HMOs is less clear. Unlike the managed-competition proposals, a *single-payer system* would replace private health insurance with federal government financing of health care. In essence, the government would assume the risk for all health care services and would pay all health care claims. Medical services would still be provided by the traditional providers – hospitals, physicians, etc. – and all medically-necessary services would be covered.

A single-payer system would be financed through payroll and other taxes. However, the effect of these new taxes would be offset by savings which employers and individuals would realize from no longer having to pay premiums for health insurance. Costs would be controlled through national and state budgets, and states would negotiate fees directly with health care providers.

While HMOs might play some role in providing care in such a system, the single-payer approach would make health insurance obsolete. As the government would take on the financial risk for health care, insurance carriers and HMOs would no longer be necessary. Single-payer proposals are the most far-reaching of the reform models and could substantially change the structure of the current system. For this reason, single-payer proposals are the least likely to be implemented without significant compromise and modification as they work their way through Congress.

Other reform proposals deal with "incremental" measures that would make minor adjustments in the operations of the existing health care system while leaving the system itself largely intact. These incremental reforms include limits on malpractice awards, caps on Medicare/Medicaid spending, and incentives and subsidies to help people buy coverage.

At this writing, the details of any ultimate legislative configuration of national health reform remain unclear. Quite aside from any legislative initiatives, however, health care reform is being driven by the market, by purchasers of health care who are demanding greater accountability, consistent quality and better value. In many states, local reform is already underway, in areas such as small group insurance, reforms of underwriting practices and increased formation of employer purchasing pools.

Federal and state legislation will play their greatest roles in determining the breadth and speed of reform – whether employers are required to provide coverage, whether universal access will be achieved and how soon. Depending on which reform model eventually gains the widest support, and its subsequent modification through the legislative process, the specific details and effects of a reformed health system may be elusive for some time to come. It appears, though, that reform has become inevitable and that HMOs will probably have an important role to play in the new reformed American health care system.

Beyond HMOs

One may rightly conclude that HMOs and managed care are complex solutions designed to correct complex problems found in the traditional health care system. As we have seen in this book, HMOs compensate for inefficiencies in the traditional health care system by adding a layer of administration to the process of delivering care. Compared to the unmanaged system, HMOs and managed care are successful because they get results – costs are lower with the same or better quality.

However, it is probably a mistake to think that HMOs are the perfect health care solution, or that they have evolved to their fullest potential. It may be most useful to think of current HMOs as a prototype for some future health care system, something that is even more efficient, even more accessible, of even higher quality and at lower cost.

Consider that the relationships between HMOs and their contracting hospitals, physician groups and other providers are sometimes adversarial. HMOs want to pay less for services while providers wish to be paid more. As a result, HMOs and providers can sometimes work at cross-purposes, instead of toward the common good of HMO members and patients. Nevertheless, in the best plan–provider relationships, these economic considerations are transcended by a mutual realization that each party is dependent on the other for success and for the common goal of delivering quality care and customer satisfaction.

These model relationships point the way toward the next phase in the evolution of health care. One can imagine a future health-care system with a means of financing that encourages all the right practices and results in all the right behaviors and outcomes. Incentives for hospitals, physicians and HMO administrators would all be aligned in the same direction – providing necessary care for the patient, efficiently and economically.

Such a system would not need the added bureaucracy of a traditional HMO to manage care, because the elements of the system would be self-managing. The additional layer of administration and expense involved in health alliances, global budgets and national health boards would not be necessary either, because incentives would result in care being appropriate, affordable and accessible to all.

In this ideal system, managed-care techniques would have become integrated into the practice of medicine so that case management would no longer be done by third parties, but rather as a natural component of good medical care. The process of care would have acquired these dimensions of managed care while returning the focus of care to its essential elements – the patient, the practitioner, and the therapeutic process.

Index